A How-to Guide

Tattoo Removal: Establishing a Free or Low-Cost Community-Based Program

By Jails to Jobs, Inc.

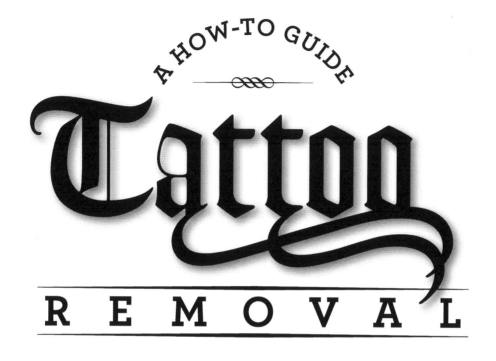

A HOW-TO GUIDE

Tattoo
REMOVAL

Establishing a
Free or Low-Cost
Community-Based
Program

JAILS TO JOBS™

Library of Congress Control Number: 2015912731
Jails to Jobs, Inc., Lafayette, CA

For further information on this book, workshops, classes and speaking engagements contact: info@jailstojobs.org

Connect with Jails to Jobs at: www.jailstojobs.org

ISBN 978-0-9912197-4-2

All of the net proceeds from the sale of this book go to Jails to Jobs, Inc., a Section 501 (c) (3) public charity, to fund its work in the creation of more free and low-cost tattoo removal programs, throughout the country, and ultimately reduce recidivism and improve public safety.

Jails to Jobs, Inc., is a member of the Global Homeboy Network.

Published by:
Jails to Jobs, Inc.
3641 Mount Diablo Blvd., #1164
Lafayette, CA 94549

Writer: Judy Jacobs
Research and Proofreading: Gary Drevno
Analysis and Publicity: Antonette Garcia
Marketing Consultant: Daniel Oxenburgh
Research: Charlene Savarino
Book Design: Ianziti Design
Project Manager: Mark Drevno

Reviewers:
Thanks and gratitude goes to each of the following individuals and their colleagues and staff for reviewing the contents of this book.

Cia Bond, *Executive Director,* Metrocrest Medical Foundation, Carrollton, Texas
Eric F. Bernstein, M.D., M.S.E., Main Line Center for Laser Surgery, Ardmore, Pa.
Fr. Greg Boyle, *Founder and Executive Director*, Homeboy Industries, Los Angeles, Calif.
Janet Allenspach, *Program Coordinator,* Liberty Tattoo Removal Program, San Luis Obispo, Calif.
Martin Hernandez, *Clinic Coordinator,* Santa Paula Tattoo Removal Program, Santa Paula, Calif.
Matthieu Vollmer, former *Marketing and Communications Coordinator,* American Society for Laser Medicine and Surgery, Wausau, Wis.
Tamara Bartlett, *Project Erase Tattoo Removal Program Coordinator,* Outside In, Portland, Ore.
William J. McClure, M.D., Napa Valley Plastic Surgery, Napa, Calif.

Table of contents

Jails to Jobs: What we do

Jails to Jobs is a Northern California based 501(c) (3) public charity that gives previously incarcerated men and women the tools they need to find employment. We conduct job search workshops for soon-to-be-released inmates in several jails and prisons in the San Francisco Bay Area.

Our website contains extensive information on topics ranging from how to write resumes and reach hiring managers to apprenticeship programs and resources for job seekers. It also includes our most current directory of more than 200 free and low-cost tattoo removal programs in 37 states that has become the most visited section of our site.

Between the popularity of that directory and our blog articles, we realized that there is a tremendous interest in the subject of anti-social and gang-related tattoo removal. That realization spurred us to create this how-to guide. The goal of this guide is to encourage more programs to support rescued victims of human trafficking, and formerly gang-involved and/or previously incarcerated men and women in order to help further their transformation and healing.

Getting visible tattoos removed—especially those that are anti-social and gang-related—should be one of the first steps people out of prison or jail should take when beginning to search for employment. Studies have shown that having these tattoos is one of the main reasons they don't get hired for jobs. And securing employment means, by some estimates, that a previously incarcerated person is 80% less likely to commit a crime and be arrested again.

We encourage you, the readers of this guide, to subscribe to our blog, like us on Facebook and follow us on Twitter, all of which can be done at www.jailstojobs.org.

Frequently asked questions

Q. **What are some of the reasons people want to get their tattoos taken off?**

Perhaps the most important reason that previously incarcerated men and women, former gang members and those who have been trafficked want their tattoos removed is to start a new life. They want to erase the reminders of their past and get back on their feet. One of the best ways to do this is to get rid of their tattoos.

For those who have decided to leave a gang, having a gang-related tattoo can be a life-or-death issue. It's possible that those people may be identified as a member of their former gang by a rival gang member and attacked or even killed.

Another very important reason to get a visible tattoo removed is so that person can gain employment and make enough money that they don't have to return to their former "career," whether it be robbery, drug dealing or burglary.

Q. **What do obstacles to employment for previously incarcerated men and women and the formerly gang-involved mean for U.S. society?**

One of the main reasons that previously incarcerated men and women are re-incarcerated is because of a lack of employment, and visible tattoos, especially those gang related or with anti-social messages, are among the biggest impediments to employment for previously incarcerated individuals, those who have been trafficked and formerly gang-involved.

Incarceration is a tremendous cost to American society—not just in wasted lives but also in the price to be paid for keeping people in prison. Although estimates vary, according to The Hamilton Project, an economic policy initiative at the Brookings Institution about $80 billion was spent on federal, state and local prisons in 2010, an increase from about $17 billion 20 years earlier.

To put things in perspective, the cost of a year at a New Jersey prison in 2011 was $44,000, while the cost of tuition for a year at Princeton University was $37,000.

Q. **Why should I—or my organization—start a free or low-cost tattoo removal program?**

Creating a free or low-cost tattoo removal program can be one of the services—or the only service— offered by a nonprofit, doctor, hospital or other organization that would like to help people turn their lives around offer.

There's an enormous need for this type of service, and, as an organization, you will be providing a tremendous benefit to society by offering it.

We discovered the need when we created a one-of-a-kind national directory of free and low-cost tattoo removal programs for our website. The directory now includes more than 200 programs, but most of them are concentrated in certain parts of the country. We have only been able to find them in 37 states. Some of these states just have a program or two, and 13 states have none at all.

Q. What are the benefits of this type of program for a community?

This type of program gives people who want to turn their lives around a chance to do so and provides a real service to the communities where they are located. Freedom from visible tattoos can transform lives. People will not only be more likely to gain employment, but once employed are less likely to return to a life of crime and prison. The programs also can divert at-risk youth from harm's way and improve public safety.

Q. How do I go about starting a program?

As outlined in this guide, there are a variety of models that can deliver a successful community-based tattoo removal program. We include different scenarios for delivering services on page 29.

One of them, for example, is connecting with a hospital, which should have practice management and other needed support services in place. The same is true if you decide to work with a local physician or other medical practitioner. In either case, you may also need volunteers for such duties as registration and case management to support the hospital or doctor's staff.

By reviewing the case studies and the tips and advice sections of this guide, as well as the forms in the appendix, you will be able to see what existing programs have determined necessary in terms of the supplies, volunteers and forms needed to operate a successful community-based program.

In most cases, a simpler, quicker way to launch a program is by following the Pop-up Program model outlined in detail on pages 30 and 31. By using this model, especially at the beginning, costs can sometimes be better managed. Fundraising conducted along the way, if necessary, can help to meet the $300-$400 per hour it costs (San Francisco Bay Area rates) to rent a machine with a nurse to do the procedures for a typical four hour session.

You can tap into service organizations such as the Rotary Club, Kiwanis, Soroptimist, church groups or a local chamber of commerce for both volunteer help and donations. Other potential fundraising options are described on page 45.

In order to understand exactly what is needed on the day of the event, you may want to contact one or more of the laser device rental companies listed on pages 38–40. They should be able to offer advice on what it takes to run a successful session, as well as subsequent future sessions that should take place at least every six to eight weeks in an ongoing program.

And remember to check out our Tattoo Removal Program Directory on pages 68–93, with the most current version at www.jailstojobs.org. It has a list of over 200 programs in 37 states. Many of them are happy to share best practices and advice on running a successful program with others who may want to start their own.

Q. Where can I recruit medical and other volunteers?

There are many places to find a variety of volunteers who might be interested in getting involved in a free- or low-cost tattoo removal program. These include:

- The health education, community education or other similar departments of hospitals.
- Local doctors, especially dermatologists and plastic surgeons, nurse practitioners, nurses and physician assistants.
- Tattoo artists.
- Professional associations. (See the list on pages 43 and 44.)
- Service clubs – Rotary, Kiwanis, Lions, Optimists, Soroptimists, HandsOn Network.
- Churches, synagogues, mosques, temples and other religious organizations.

Q. Why would a doctor or medical professional want to volunteer in a tattoo-removal program or even start one from scratch?

In our experience, members of the medical profession can be very caring and compassionate people. In many cases a desire to serve and heal others is what brought them to medicine in the first place.

We feel that it's not necessary to try to convince or persuade a prospective volunteer to get involved. In fact, that might be counterproductive. Instead, organizations can publicize the opportunity in their communities and allow those interested to come forward.

Please also see item No. 7 in Pop-up Program Model section on page 30 of our guide. It includes the benefits that teaching hospitals can gain by offering such a program.

These programs are considered newsworthy, and it is not unusual for physicians and other healthcare professionals who volunteer in them to be mentioned in newspaper and magazine articles or professional association newsletters or journals. This can bring recognition from colleagues and opportunities to expand one's medical practice.

There are volunteer tattoo removal practitioners who are amazingly committed to the mission of the organizations they work with. One doctor flies from Massachusetts to Los Angeles to volunteer at Homeboy Industries' tattoo removal program for one week every month.

Q. How much will it cost, and how can I pay for it?

There are a variety of ways to do this, and the case study section of this guide gives examples of how a few organizations and individuals have created and managed to fund these programs. In many cases they cost nothing to the organization, since all of the services and supplies are donated.

Some programs are funded by cities or counties, often as part of gang-prevention efforts. Others charge fees, but the cost is far less than what it would be if the person were to go to a private doctor to have their tattoos removed.

In hospital programs, the procedures are usually done by staff physicians and the supplies donated by the hospital. In one case study we include, the founder of a private organization paid the cost of the equipment and the program out-of-pocket but uses the money he earns from full-paying clients to help fund his program.

Q. Who is qualified to do the removals?

People with all sorts of qualifications do tattoo removals. They may be doctors, nurse practitioners, physician assistants, nurses, aestheticians, tattoo artists or someone who took training just to do them.

It's crucial to be aware of the fact, however, that tattoo removal programs are regulated on a state-by-state basis, and each state has different laws. In some states the procedure is considered to be the practice of medicine and subject to the same types of laws that regulate other medical procedures. In a handful of states, a physician is required to be at the facility during the procedure.

We're not aware of any resource that includes the laws relating to tattoo removal for each state, so the best thing to do is to contact the medical board and the board of registered nursing of the state in which you are located. A list of these can be found on the website of New Look Laser College at: http://newlooklasercollege.com/tattoo-removal-training/who-can-perform.

Q. What equipment is necessary?

Tattoo removal practitioners, in most cases, use a Q-switched laser device. There are descriptions of the types of devices and the companies that sell them on pages 32–36.

Q. How do I get the equipment?

You can buy it directly from the company or purchase it used, if you'd like to have your own device. Another options is to rent the equipment, either alone or with a nurse or technician to perform the procedures.

Q. What if I want to learn how to do the procedures myself?

Although most tattoo removal procedures are done by medical professionals, we know of tattoo artists who do them and of at least one dedicated person—his story is included in our case studies—who went out and learned how to perform tattoo removals himself. There is a directory of schools that teach how to do it on pages 41 and 42.

Q. Is it a good idea to partner with other organizations and people to provide additional services?

Yes, it definitely can be, since many previously incarcerated people, formerly gang-involved individuals or those who have been trafficked need help with a lot of issues besides tattoo removal.

Some organizations partner with other groups and individuals to sponsor a free or low-cost tattoo removal clinic that also includes information about housing, GED programs, resume writing, health care and other community services that may be of interest to those who come to get their tattoos taken off.

Tattoo and tattoo removal facts

The problems of visible tattoos

- A Harris Poll of 2,016 adults surveyed online between Jan. 16 and 23, 2012 found that:
  - 14% of those who have gotten a tattoo regretted it later.
  - 27% of respondents said that people with tattoos are less intelligent, and 25% said they are less healthy.

- A survey of 2,878 hiring managers conducted by Harris Interactive for CareerBuilder in early 2011 found that 37% of respondents said they would be less likely to hire someone with visible tattoos, the third reason after only piercings and bad breath. (In the case that these tattoos are gang- or drug-related or anti-social the percentage may be much higher.)

- Human trafficking ranks as the globe's fastest growing criminal industry, earning perpetrators an estimated $32 billion each year. Girls and women who are trafficked for prostitution are often tattooed by their pimp—with his name, gang tag, a dollar sign or even a barcode—declaring to the world that they are the pimp's property. These tattoos can be found on various parts of the body, including the neck, arms, legs, faces, breasts, eyelids and even, in some cases, their gums.

- University of West Virginia Ph.D. candidate Kaitlyn Harger's research found that people with visible tattoos who were released from prisons and jails were re-incarcerated about one-third more quickly than those without visible tattoos.

- The military is tightening restrictions on tattoos, and branches limit what tattoos say, as well as their location on a person's body and/or size.

Taking them off

- American Society of Dermatologic Surgery—member doctors performed roughly 100,000 tattoo-removal procedures in 2011, the latest year for which statistics are available. It was a 16.3% increase over the previous year's figure of 86,000.

- Although there are a variety of tattoo removal methods—including dermabrasion, which removes the outer layers of the skin—the most common is a medical procedure using Q-switched laser devices.

- The number of sessions needed to remove a tattoo by using a Q-switched laser devise can vary from two to ten or more.

- The time between tattoo removal treatments is usually six to eight weeks.

- The Kirby Desai Scale, created by two osteopathic doctors, William Kirby and Alpesh Desai, and published in the March 2009 edition of the Journal of Clinical and Aesthetic Dermatology, measures the difficulty of removing a particular tattoo.

- Factors determining ease of removal of a particular tattoo include the color(s) of the tattoo, how long ago it was done, whether it was done by a professional or amateur tattoo artist, and where on the body it is located.

- Low-cost or free tattoo removal programs take a wide variety of forms. These include nonprofits that recruit volunteer doctors and staffs, hospital-sponsored programs, pop-up programs, mobile units and pre-release programs operated by prison, sheriff's or probation departments.

Tattoos through time: A brief history

The art of tattooing has been around for millennia and practiced by people just about everywhere in the world. Whether a tribal tattoo recognizing a warrior's success in battle or a rose adorning a modern-day millennial, tattoos have been a distinctive form of self-expression—and, in some cases, a badge of dishonor—throughout the ages.

The first example of tattooing was found on a mummy named Amunent, a fertility priestess who is thought to have lived sometime between 4000 BCE and 4160 BCE, and another female mummy thought to have been a dancer. Because of the erotic nature of these early tattoos, archaeologists believe that in the earliest days only women wore them.

Another example of a mummy sporting tattoos is the so-called Otzi the Iceman, discovered in 1991 in the Alps near the border of Austria and Italy. Otzi, who archaeologists estimate lived between 3350 BCE and 3100 BCE, had more than 50 tattoos consisting of lines and crosses. Scientists were amazed when they realized that the tattoos, made by rubbing charcoal into skin incisions, corresponded to certain acupuncture points in Chinese medicine where his body would have experienced stress and strain from the lifestyle he led. Therefore, it is believed that, rather than purely decorative, these tattoos may have been a form of therapy.

Peruvian mummy reveals extensive tattoos

The legs, arms and feet of a female mummy—discovered in a Peruvian pyramid at an ancient site known as El Brujo—were covered with tattoos of spiders, snakes and other animals. Based on the significance of the items found buried with her, she is believed to have been an important person. No one knows, however, the type of role she played in the ancient Moche civilization that ruled the northern coastal area of Peru during the period of 100 CE to 800 CE.

Meanwhile, writings at the time indicate that various central and northern European tribes in the pre-Christian era sported tattoos. In ancient China, tattoos were mainly found on the bodies of bandits, and the faces of criminals were forcefully tattooed to display their status.

Throughout other parts of Asia, tattoos were most common among the indigenous tribal peoples, many of whom continue the practice to this day, although it is dying out with the young generation. In the Philippines, the Bontoc people of northern Luzon are noted for their tattoos, the practice of which, as in the case of other indigenous peoples, arose to celebrate successes at headhunting.

The Iban people who live in longhouses scattered through the jungles of Malaysian and Indonesian Borneo, traditionally covered their upper bodies with tattoos depicting plants, animals and life experiences. Another tribe of longhouse dwellers along the Rajang River in Malaysian Borneo, the Kayan, were known for tattooing their young girls' hands, upper feet and later other parts of their bodies.

The Polynesian people of the Pacific islands also had a tattoo tradition, which has been in existence for two millennia. The word "tattoo," in fact, comes from the Tahitian "tatau," which was first documented in the west by the naturalist aboard Captain James Cook's ship, *The Endeavor*.

Although there are many shared elements, the people of French Polynesia, Samoa, New Zealand (Maoris) and Hawaii had their own styles, applied by needles made from such natural elements as bamboo, bird bone or even shark's teeth.

Body ink in the Americas and beyond

Among other indigenous cultures around the world that practiced tattooing are the Ainu of Japan, who tattooed their teenage girls as a rite of passage. Many tribes in the Amazon region of South America are noted for tattooing their faces, along with other parts of their bodies. The Matis, Marubo and Kayabi are among the few groups that continue the practice today.

In North America, tattooing was practiced among some American Indian tribes, a custom noted in the writings of explorers and the early Jesuit missionaries. The Iroquois tattooed themselves with symbols that identified the clan to which they belonged. Women of the Cree tribe were tattooed with facial lines, while the men covered a greater area of their bodies.

During the 18th century, French sailors came back from the South Pacific sporting tattoos, creating an interest in them in Europe. Members of the British Navy began a tattooing tradition a century later.

In the United States, the military has a long history of tattooing, begun in the early 19th century by members of the U.S. Navy who returned from far-away lands, where they had encountered tattoo-wearing cultures. The practice became entrenched, and through the World Wars and onward, military members got tattoos to mark their units, the battles they fought in or an occasional romantic interest they picked up along the way.

More recently, tattoos have entered the popular culture, and everyone from gang members to the lawyers who represent them may have body ink. It would be next to impossible to spend a few hours on the streets of any major city in the U.S. and not see someone sporting a tattoo of some type.

Although many people get their tattoos done with (hopefully) sterilized equipment in tattoo shops, those in jail or prison get primitive tattoos usually made using homemade tattoo guns put together with items that are likely to include a pen, wire, a toothbrush and a motor. The ink may be made from melted checker or chess pieces, ink pen caps, soot or other things.

Who's tattooed: Study shows numbers, attitudes

In recent decades, tattoos have become a popular means of self-expression and can be found adorning the bodies of people of all ages. It is estimated, in fact, that 21%—or about one in five—of U.S. adults has at least one tattoo. This number is up from 14% of adults in 2008.

A Harris Poll of 2,016 adults surveyed online between Jan. 16 and 23, 2012 found that tattoos are more prevalent among certain age groups.

Although one might think that it's the young 20-somethings that are getting most of the tattoos, that's simply not the case. According to the Harris Poll results, tattoos are most prevalent among adults aged 30 to 39–38% of this group has a tattoo—while just 30% of those between the ages of 25 and 29 and 22% of those between 18 and 24 have one. The numbers for older Americans: 27% of those between 40 and 49 years of age, 11% of those between 50 and 64, and just 5% of those 65 and older have body art.

Beyond age, there are regional differences in numbers of residents sporting tattoos. Tattoos seem to be most prevalent in the West—26% of adults in that region report having at least one—compared to fewer in the East with 21%, the Midwest also with 21% and the South with18%.

Although it may come as a surprise to some, women are slightly more likely than men to be tattooed—23% of women versus 19% of men overall.

Attitudes rule

While the poll found that only 14% of those who had gotten a tattoo regretted it later, the attitudes of people without tattoos, who were also among those interviewed, revealed how society views body ink.

Here is their opinion:

- At least two respondents out of five said that people with tattoos are less attractive (45%) or sexy (39%).
- One-quarter said that people with tattoos are less intelligent (27%), healthy (25%) or spiritual (25%).
- Half of those without a tattoo said that people with tattoos are more rebellious (50%).

More people want them off

Although tattoos are removed by nurses, nurse practitioners, physician assistants, and tattoo technicians as well as doctors, the statistics that come from the American Society of Dermatologic Surgery (ASDS) may give an overall picture of a growing interest among people with tattoos who want to get them removed.

ASDS-member doctors performed roughly 100,000 tattoo-removal procedures in 2011, the latest year for which statistics are available. It was a 16.3% increase over the previous year's figure of 86,000.

Victims of human trafficking and abuse desperate to erase their past

Although most Americans are totally unaware of its existence here in the U.S., human trafficking is a horrendous crime that is happening right on the streets of our cities and in many of our neighborhoods. In fact, it ranks as the globe's fastest growing criminal industry, earning perpetrators an estimated $32 billion each year.

While the press often focuses on foreigners as human trafficking victims (even in this country), a study analyzing U.S. Dept. of Justice Human Trafficking Task Force cases found that 83% of sex trafficking victims in the U.S. are actually U.S. citizens.

Trafficked individuals might be forced into servitude doing agricultural, restaurant, household, factory or other work without getting paid. The majority of victims, however, are forced participants in the commercial sex industry, where the average age of those first victimized ranges from 12 to 14 years of age.

Many of these young people are runaways, who get caught up in the trade because they need money to live and are taken advantage of. The places they're most likely to be "recruited" are homeless shelters and shopping malls. Another way criminals find young people to traffick is through social media.

Once trafficked, it's difficult, if not impossible, for them to escape. To prevent them from getting away, they may be accompanied in public by a controlling "boyfriend," who is actually their pimp. As awareness of this problem becomes more widespread, a growing number of organizations and task forces across the country are working to free these young people from sexual slavery.

Victims of sex trafficking are often tattooed by their pimp with his name, gang tag, a dollar sign or even a barcode declaring to the world that they are the pimp's property. These tattoos can be found on various parts of the body, including the neck, arms, legs, faces, breasts, eyelids and even, in some cases, their gums. Removing this type of tattoo can be a major step in the recovery process, once victims are rescued, and can help restore their dignity and self-esteem.

Pimps are not the only people who force tattoos on people they control. Some women in sexually and/ or psychologically abusive relationships are forcibly tattooed by their husbands or boyfriends, often with the man's name to remind them who "owns" them. Once the woman breaks free from the relationship, removing the tattoo can be a major step to erase a visible sign of her past and help in the healing process.

It's important for doctors and healthcare workers to be aware of what to look for—barcode tattoos and tattoos with a man's name or a weird symbol that the wearer cannot explain, or a controlling "boyfriend" who comes to appointment, among other signs—to determine whether someone might be the victim of human trafficking.

To learn more about human trafficking, please visit www.traffickingresourcecenter.org.

Tattoos create barriers at work and elsewhere

While many people who get tattoos may feel that it's a cool thing to do, they may have not been thinking too seriously about the consequences of their actions.

Those with tattoos can face a variety of obstacles, from having difficulty finding a job or getting promoted to being identified as a member of a gang they no longer belong to. They may also find themselves limited in their choice of mates or rejected by the military, among other things.

Hiring managers may not be amused

While attitudes among the general public toward people with tattoos tend not to be particularly favorable, even more important may be the attitudes of hiring managers. Although much on the subject is anecdotal, a study at Bowling Green State University in Ohio cited in a May 2013 article on the Society for Industrial & Organizational Psychology website offers insight into the preconceived notions that those who hire may have about applicants with body ink.

Doctoral student Ryan Wharton and psychology professor Scott Highhouse conducted research on the influence that tattoos played in hiring decisions. A research sample of hiring managers were each given a single resume, but a varied job description—one for a help desk and the other for a call-center position. They also received a photo of one of five men with different types of tattoos applied by computer photo editing.

A questionnaire found that the managers would not be interested in hiring anyone with more than one tattoo, even if that person would not be working with the public.

A survey of 2,878 hiring managers conducted by Harris Interactive for CareerBuilder in early 2011 found that visible tattoos were the third personal attribute that would make employers less likely to promote an employee, after piercings and bad breath. Of those surveyed, 37% said they would be less likely to hire someone with piercings, 34% for those with bad breath and 31% for those with visible tattoos.

You're in the army now—or not

The Army does not allow tattoos on the face, head, scalp or neck above the Class A shirt collar. It had loosened its rules on tattoos in 2006 to allow tattoos that were not racist, sexist or in other ways offensive on the hands. Officials are about to change that, however, restricting all tattoos to above the knees and elbows and below the neckline.

The Navy has similar restrictions regarding tattoos on the face, head, scalp and neck and does not allow tattoos anywhere that are sexually explicit, obscene or advocate discrimination or indicate affiliation with a gang, or supremacist or extremist group.

In addition to a prohibition on head and neck tattoos, members of the U.S. Marine Corps. cannot be tattooed on their hands, fingers, wrists or inside of their mouths. Commissioned and warrant officers are only allowed four tattoos that can be seen when they wear the standard physical training uniform, and these tattoos can be no larger than the wearer's outstretched hand.

The U.S. Air Force website is not as clear about tattoo restrictions as the other service branches, but it does say that tattoos that are obscene or advocate discrimination are prohibited and that excessive tattoos—those covering more than 25% of a particular body part—are not allowed. It also says that anyone with any questions on the subject can chat with an Air Force online advisor or get in touch with their local recruiter.

Even tattoo artists find practice questionable

Perhaps few people are more informed about the impact of body ink than tattoo artists, and no one has a more vested interest in seeing more people tattooed. It's their livelihood, after all.

Karen Hudson is one person who should know. One of the world's top body art acceptance advocates for more than a decade, the author of *"Living Canvas: Your Total Guide to Tattoos, Piercings, and Body Modification"* and the editor of *"Chick Ink: 40 Stories of Tattoo—and the Women Who Wear Them,"* she also served a year as an apprentice in a tattoo studio and displays more than her share of body art herself.

In an article on about.com, she writes that many studios have policies that prevent them from doing visible tattoos—tattoos on hands, feet or, most importantly, faces. According to her, that for tattoo artists it's a moral issue, since they are quite well aware of the difficulties people with visible tattoos may face in the job market and in their personal and professional lives.

These tattoo artists feel a certain sense of responsibility towards their clients and potential clients to ensure that these people don't make irresponsible decisions they are likely to regret later on.

The effect of tattoo removal on recidivism rates

About 70% of those released from prison each year are tattooed. The stigma of visible tattoos—those located on the arms, hands, neck or face of an individual—can present serious problems for those in reentry as they search for employment. In fact, previously incarcerated individuals with visible tattoos go back to prison 714 days sooner than previously incarcerated men and women with nonvisible tattoos. According to The Economist this acceleration of recidivism translates into an extra cost of $5.5 billion per year to U.S. taxpayers.

Research done by Jake Cronin of the University of Missouri, Harry S. Truman School of Public Policy, indicates that the probability of a previously incarcerated individual returning to prison is 61% greater if that person is not employed fulltime. Removing gang-related and anti-social tattoos dramatically increases a person's ability to attain employment.

Additional research on this subject was conducted by Kaitlyn Harger, a PhD candidate in economics at the University of West Virginia. In a paper entitled, "Bad Ink: Visible Tattoos and Recidivism," Harger examines whether visible tattoos affect recidivism rates. She used data from the Florida Department of Corrections Offender Based Information System to compare the amount of time that those displaying visible tattoos were able to remain out of prison with the amount of time for those with no tattoos or tattoos that could be covered up by clothing.

The data was for all inmates released from Florida facilities during 2008, 2009 and 2010—a total of 97,156 people, with 88% of the sample male, 50% white, 46% black and 3.6% Hispanic. It included not just such demographic data as gender, race and age, and a list of offenses, but also information on the type and body location of each of the inmates' tattoos. While 22% of Harger's sample population had visible tattoos on their head, face, neck or hands, 63% had them on any of those places plus their arms or legs. Arm and leg tattoos would be visible if the person was wearing a T-shirt or shorts, which might be the case in certain jobs, including that of construction worker and lifeguard.

What Harger found was that the expected length of time between release and re-incarceration for inmates with tattoos in general was 32.4% less than those without tattoos. And the expected length of time between release and re-incarceration for those with tattoos on the head, face, back or hands was 27.4% less than those with tattoos in other places.

Kevin Waters' research in a paper titled, "The Tattooed Inmate and Recidivism," offered evidence that previously incarcerated individuals with visible tattoos are more likely to commit felony offenses and new violent offenses for which they are reconvicted within three years of their release. From his research, Waters believes that laser tattoo removal should be made readily available to soon-to-be released prisoners as a pre-release offering. "The purpose of tattoo removal would serve to symbolically disaffiliate the inmate from gangs or prison primary groups while enhancing post-release employment opportunities," he says. Unfortunately, tattoo removal programs for adult prisoners are virtually nonexistent in the United States. We have only been able to find five such programs.

Regardless of the reason, visible tattoos are costing states and the Federal government a tremendous amount of money. In the case of Florida, previously incarcerated individuals with visible tattoos return to prison 419 days earlier than those without. At $47.50, the average daily price of housing an inmate, it would cost an additional $19,903 per year per inmate with a visible tattoo or a total of about $418 million over the three-year time period that Harger studied. The Vera Institute of Justice analysis concludes the average annual cost of housing one prisoner in the United States is $31,286.

David O. Carter, United States District Court Judge for the Central District of California, has stated that previously incarcerated men and women who get their tattoos taken off "gain a much needed boost in confidence and self-esteem. By having tattoos removed, they would not be pre-judged, and they would be better able to communicate and get a job." In referring to the U.S. District Court's Offender Tattoo Removal Program, he went on to say, "This program has saved Orange County (Calif.) millions of dollars because for every $1 it costs for the tattoo removal program, it costs $7 for incarceration." He is hopeful that this program will serve as a model for the entire country.

In most cases, it appears community-based tattoo removal programs measure their success through anecdotal means. However, Community Action Partnership's Liberty Tattoo Removal Program, established in 2000 in San Luis Obispo, Calif., tracks its results and offers very encouraging data for previously incarcerated individuals that have removed their visible tattoos. Sixty percent of its clients are parolees who have just a 10% recidivism rate, compared with the California state average of 70% according to the organization's report.

In all cases employers are quite outspoken with their disapproval of visible tattoos—61% of human resource managers believe a visible tattoo damages a job applicant's chances of gaining employment. "The influence of appearance goes beyond the hiring process. It has an impact on the perception of one's competence," say the authors of an annual study on professionalism in the workplace from the Centre for Professional Excellence at York College of Pennsylvania.

Taking 'em off

Getting a tattoo removed can be a long and painful process, but how long and how painful depends on a variety of factors.

There are a number of ways to remove tattoos employed over the years. Most of these procedures have been replaced by the Q-switched laser device, but some of them are still utilized on occasion.

In one of these methods known as salabration, a salt solution is applied to scrub the tattoo away. Scarring is a potential side effect, and this method is not only ineffective at removing tattoos but also no longer very common.

Tricholoracetic acid (TCA), a process also known as a chemical peel or controlled burn, is still sold and used by people who try to remove their own tattoos. Like salabration, this technique hasn't proved very effective, since the acid doesn't go deep enough into the skin to remove all of the tattoo pigment.

Dermabrasion, which removes the outer layers of the skin, is still performed by some plastic surgeons to remove tattoos. They apply a local anesthetic and then liquid nitrogen, before using a sanding tool or other device to remove the top layers of skin, and hopefully the tattoo.

According to the American Society for Dermatologic Surgery, some patients may choose this option because it could cost less than laser surgery and has been done for many years. Like laser surgery, however, dermabrasion requires a series of treatments, and those who have it done must avoid direct sunlight for three to six months afterwards to prevent scarring.

Another method still used is a procedure known as surgical excision, in which the tattoo is actually cut out and the surrounding skin stitched together under local anesthetic. The advantage of this method is that it can be done in one session. The disadvantage is that it can only be performed on small tattoos and may cause scarring, always something to be considered.

Q-switched laser devices

Since Q-switched lasers were introduced commercially in the early 1990s, they have become the preferred method of tattoo removal. This technique uses a laser beam to break up the dye pigment, which is then flushed away by the body. Some colors, like black, are easier to break up, because they absorb all of the laser wavelengths. Other colors prove more difficult because they don't absorb certain wavelengths.

Laser treatment is tailored to each patient and will depend on a lot of things, including whether the tattoo was done by a professional tattoo artist or an amateur, like those done in prisons; how long ago the patient got the tattoo; the size of the tattoo; the patient's skin color; and how deep the tattoo ink has penetrated into the layers of skin.

A laser, which actually stands for Light Amplification by the Stimulated Emission of Radiation, produces single wavelengths of light in a series of pulses that lasts just nanoseconds or as a narrow beam. It targets certain colors of ink with the wavelength of light that works best to remove those colors. It's essential to apply that wavelength with the correct amount of power and for exactly the right amount of time to ensure success.

Picosecond laser devices

The latest technology for tattoo removal was pioneered by researchers more than a decade and a half ago but has become commercially available in more recent years. That technology, picosecond laser pulses, is incorporated in picosecond Q-switched lasers and employs extremely short pulses—shorter than those produced by the nanosecond Q-switched lasers that are still the most commonly used devices currently on the market.

Proponents of picosecond lasers say that the technique is more effective and requires fewer treatments but they are not able to treat the full spectrum of tattoo ink colors.

Kirby Desai Scale

The length of time it takes to remove a tattoo can vary from four sessions to many more than that. The number of sessions necessary used to be nearly impossible to predict, but two osteopathic doctors, William Kirby and Alpesh Desai, created what is known as the Kirby Desai Scale. This is the first ever means of being able to measure the difficulty of removing a particular tattoo on a scale of 4 to 26.

They published their findings in the March 2009 edition of the Journal of Clinical and Aesthetic Dermatology, and some tattoo removal practitioners have started to use the scale to estimate the number of treatments needed and the potential cost for the patient.

To determine the number of treatments necessary to remove a particular tattoo, the practitioner gives a numerical value to six different aspects of the patient and their tattoo—the location, amount of ink, color, person's skin type, layering and scarring. Those six numbers are then added together.

According to Kirby and Desai, if a patient and their tattoo have a score of more than 15, they might want to reconsider with their physician whether they want it removed, because it will be quite difficult to do so.

Whatever the score, tattoo removal treatment sessions should be scheduled about six to eight weeks apart. When there's less time between sessions, scarring is more likely to occur.

Factors determining ease of removal

There are a wide variety of factors beyond color that makes some tattoos more difficult to remove than others. Some of these include:

- Age of tattoo: The older the better, because if you have had the tattoo longer it is more likely to fade.

- Tattoo artist who did it: Tattoos done by amateurs are usually easier to take off than those done by professionals. Amateur tattoo artists for the most part just create tattoos in black with less pigment applied, and that pigment is not applied as deeply as it would be by a professional.

- Where it is located on a patient's body: Tattoos located on body extremities such as hands and ankles take longer to fade.

- Tattoo colors: Some colors fade better than others. Black and dark green are said to be the easiest to fade, while turquoise, yellow and fluorescent inks are the most difficult. Dark inks are easier to fade, because they are more adept at absorbing laser energy.

Pain control during the removal process

Getting tattoos removed can be a rather painful experience, compared by many to having rubber bands snapped against your skin. There are measures providers can take to help alleviate the pain, however.

The most common method is numbing cream that is rubbed on the area a certain amount of time before the procedure is done.

Although it may not be an option for most nonprofit programs, laser device manufacturer Astanza sells a skin numbing device that blows very cold air—as low as 30 degrees—over the area to help minimize the pain.

Success stories

Getting a tattoo removed can sometimes make a huge difference in the lives of those who have them. In some cases, especially when a person is trying to leave a gang or has encounters with a rival gang, a tattoo can be a life-threatening display of misplaced loyalty.

We wanted to include a few of the many stories of people who have had tattoos removed and what it has meant to them. We'd like to thank the programs that shared these stories with us. The names of their clients have all been changed to protect their privacy.

From Project Erase in Portland, Ore., comes a series of tales of tattoo removals in progress.

Erik

Erik has come in to get five tattoos removed, two of which are gang-related. He feels that the removal will help him lead a more "positive, safe, and healthy lifestyle." The process is going well. He had two on his hands that had been removed at Project Erase previously, and some of the ones he's working on now will soon be gone.

He got the tattoos to show loyalty to his gang—as a means of "branding himself"—he says. Erik wanted to change his life and "didn't need to carry the tattoos around as a reminder" of his past. He feels that the process will definitely lead to more employment opportunities, because people will not be aware of his previous gang membership.

Raymond

Raymond was a drug, weapon and contraband trafficker in the Golden Triangle of Southeast Asia and a coyote when he was 14 or 15 years old in the mid-1970s. He is removing a large tattoo on his chest and shoulder that he got to fit into the social hierarchy and to keep from getting killed for disloyalty. It was a very harsh and dangerous environment.

He has never been able to publicly reveal the tattoo on his chest and shoulder for fear that he would be harmed. Raymond had one tattoo on his hand removed at a traditional removal clinic after arriving back in the U.S. He was unable to get a job because it was so visible. Removing this second tattoo is a further effort to protect his personal safety.

Tom

Tom said that the removal process is going terrifically and that he's really happy the program exists. Recently released from a correctional facility, he wants to get his tattoo removed in an effort to get out of his old lifestyle and is doing it in combination with relocating and making other changes in his life at the urging of his parole officer.

The tattoo currently being removed was from a time when he was homeless and had a meth problem. Tom was working for a gang, and they gave him the tattoo when they asked him to join. Later he was arrested for stealing a car and taking off on a high-speed chase. While in prison, Tom got into fights over his tattoo and gang affiliation. Now he is sober and out of the gang lifestyle but still has the tattoo. Because gang members have threatened to cut the tattoo off his back, Tom decided it would be better to get it removed.

After going through three treatments, Tom has noticed the tattoo fading, and with the tattoo gone, he will feel safer and more separated from his old lifestyle.

These stories come from the Community Action Partnership of San Luis Obispo County's Liberty Tattoo Removal Program in California:

Steve

Steve came to the program with a large tattoo on his neck that read SHADOW. He was unable to get a decent paying job, and the only work he could find was detailing cars at a car dealership. His previous incarceration served as another hindrance in his job search.

As his neck tattoo disappeared, Steve's attitude brightened. He enjoyed his volunteer work, and his girlfriend was feeling more positive about their future. When his tattoo was almost gone, the manager of the car dealership let him try out sales in the car showroom. Due to his almost invisible tattoo and his eager and pleasant demeanor, Steve sold enough cars in one week to break sales records for the luxury car dealership. His girlfriend accepted his proposal, they got married and moved into their own apartment together. This could never have happened if he hadn't had his visible tattoo removed.

Curtis

Curtis presented himself as a depressed, mentally disabled, homeless client with many anti-social tattoos, as well as scarring from his previous cutting behavior. His neck was covered with a slit ("cut here") and a blood tattoo dripping down. He was sullen, anti-social, dressed entirely in black and often smelled like he hadn't taken a bath in quite a while.

He began volunteering for his tattoo removal clinic requirement at the Prado Day Center, and they assisted him in getting involved with Transitions Mental Health. Diagnosed bipolar, Curtis began taking medication and continued to come to the program so that his many violent and unhappy tattoos, beginning with the one on his neck, would be removed. His personality began to lighten and improve, and he began participating in self-help services. Disability insurance came through, and Curtis received a housing voucher from Transitions Mental Health Assn. The voucher will allow him to be able to move into his first home in many years, which he hopes to find close to the shelter so that he can continue to volunteer. He wrote in a satisfaction survey that "volunteering when I'm sad makes me feel happy."

Lisa

While success stories usually come at the end of receiving service, this one came with enrollment. As a teenager, Lisa had been hooked on drugs and used as a sex-slave by an older man. Among other things, he had his name tattooed on her as a "property" mark. Several years later, this same man was convicted of murdering another female.

The day she was admitted to the program, Lisa cried and nearly collapsed because she was so grateful to have the opportunity to erase her terrible and terrifying past and begin the road to healing. She says that being in the program helped her deal with anxiety and other mental/emotional health issues that resulted from her trauma. She has had the tattoos from her previous life removed, graduated from college and is living a happy, calm existence.

Here are some more stories from the D-Tag Tattoo Removal Program of the Metrocrest Medical Foundation in Carrollton, Texas.

John

John was abused, his father was an alcoholic, and his mother left him. He wound up on the streets and in prison multiple times for theft, including one two-year stay, after which, in his late 20s, he entered the program. It took him four and a half years to get his tattoos off.

During that time, John attended junior college and mentored other young people who were in difficult situations. He received a scholarship to finish his education at Southern Methodist University, graduated summa cum laude and got another scholarship for a master's degree. John now works doing business strategy for a financial company in Dallas, owns his own marketing company and has developed IT programs for healthcare. Married to a woman who has a master's degree in nursing, he is expecting his second child.

Barry

In his mid-50s and currently in the program, Barry was in prison for quite a while and was referred to D-Tag by someone in the church where he participates in a Bible study group. Barry has full body tattoos and was beaten up because some of them are gang-related prison tattoos that were recognized by a former fellow prisoner. D-Tag is helping him get them taken off for his own safety. Barry has been able to get a job and is preparing for a better tattoo-free life.

Julia

Julia was in a community gang when she was in high school, but realized early on that she wanted a different life from the one she had had so far. In order to get that different life, she would have to get her tattoos removed. Julia wanted to go into the military but knew that wouldn't be possible with her visible tattoos. The process took three years, but it was well worth it. Julia has been in the Marines for eight years and now serves in its police force. She plans to continue to make that branch of the military her career.

From Chicago's Ink 180 Ministry comes the story of a victim of human trafficking:

Nicole

Nicole's entire life was filled with sexual abuse. Her mother sold her to pedophiles when she was 5 or 6 years old. She ran away from home at 13 and was sold by a pimp, who forced her to get a tattoo of his name on the side of her neck. After being rescued by the FBI, who called Ink 180, her pimp was sentenced to life in prison.

While being trafficked, Nicole gave birth to three children. Although her background was horrendous, she turned her life around. Not only is she a fantastic mom and involved in her church, but Nicole earned a high school diploma, graduated from college and is now a counselor working with other people who have been trafficked. In addition, she often does public speaking engagements to bring attention to the problem of human trafficking.

Questions programs may be asked

When considering setting up a tattoo removal program, you may want to also think ahead about the types of questions potential clients might ask. That way you not only can prepare to answer them but can also create a program that will meet people's needs.

Here are some things that people may ask you about your program and the tattoo removal process:

What sort of training and how much experience does the person doing the procedure have?

Anyone can take a two- to three-day course to learn to do tattoo removals, but in many states, tattoo removal is considered the practice of medicine, and some require a doctor to be on site when procedures are performed. Others don't have any regulations to that effect.

What sort of laser equipment do you use?

There are many Q-switched lasers at various price points, and some of them only remove certain colors of ink. Only the advanced lasers remove all colors, so if someone has a multi-color tattoo, they'll need the more advanced equipment.

How good are your results?

Most tattoo removal practitioners keep before-and-after photos of the procedures they've performed, so potential clients can get an idea of what type of results they can expect to get.

Although most people have hopefully done their homework, they might also ask questions about the process itself, including:

- **How does the laser work?** Having a simple easy-to-understand explanation about how lasers work to allay the fears of those who may be afraid of medical procedures could be helpful.

- **How many treatments will it take to remove my tattoo(s)?** That question can only be answered after the person doing the tattoo removal can assess each person's tattoos.

- **How many weeks do you recommend between treatments?** Most tattoo removal practitioners recommend six to eight weeks between treatments, but each program may have its own policy.

- **How much will it cost?** Each program will have its own requirements. These requirements will cover specifics such as who qualifies for free or low-cost tattoo removal and the cost of procedures, if there are any.

Different models for delivering services

Nonprofit organizations, government agencies or private doctors, nurses or others who are exploring the possibility of providing free or low-cost tattoo removal have a variety of models to rely upon.

These include:

- **Renting a laser device (nurse/technician can be included)** from one of the laser rental companies included in this guide makes it an easy point of entry.

- **Partnering with an existing program.** An example of this, Removing Barriers in San Pablo, Calif., one of the case studies included in this guide, has partnered with New Skin Adult Tattoo Removal, a community organization in San Jose.

- **Hospital-sponsored program.** These can be found throughout the country, and one example, at the Metrocrest Hospital Authority (MHA) in Carrollton, Texas, is included in our case study section.

- **Owning or leasing equipment and recruiting local doctors.** Homeboy Industries is an excellent example of this, and a description of their program can be found among our case studies.

- **Partnering with a doctor**—dermatologist, plastic surgeon or other specialist—who has a laser device and is willing to volunteer to do removals on weekends or evenings. Santa Paula Tattoo Removal Program in our case studies is an example of this.

- **Partnering with a medical aesthetician practice** like 2nd Chance Grace, one of our case study organizations, did.

- **Creating a mobile program** with an RV turned into a clinic. Ink 180, an organization based in Oswego, Ill., a Chicago suburb, launched a mobile tattoo program in the spring of 2014 with a van and two retired ambulances. Volunteers travel with one or more of these vehicles throughout inner city Chicago each week to do tattoo removals at churches and other organizations.

- **Establishing a pre-release program** through a sheriff's or probation department or a youth authority. Examples of these we are aware of are the Los Angeles County Sheriff's Department, Travis County Jail, Chicago's Cook County Jail, Kern County Probation Department and Oregon Youth Authority.

- **Establishing a church-based program** with a volunteer doctor, as did one of our case study organizations, Agape Light Tattoo Removal Program.

- **Charging market rate or discounted prices to those who can afford it**, which will help support a program. Two examples of this in our case studies are Houston Laser Institute and Taboo Tattoo Removal Program.

Pop-up program model

Organizations that would like to establish a program but can't afford to buy their own equipment can consider what we like to call the pop-up model.

The pop-up tattoo removal program model is similar to a pop-up restaurant or pop-up shop that appears for a brief time—or sometimes on a regular schedule—in a space that at other times may be used for something else. These programs can be offered regularly at a hospital, school, church, club or government building.

In the case of a tattoo removal program, an organization could establish a pop-up program in a variety of ways. Here are some examples:

1. Recruit a volunteer doctor, nurse practitioner, physician assistant, nurse or tattoo removal technician (some esthetician skin care businesses and tattoo shops offer tattoo removal) who does tattoo removal procedures as part of their regular practice or work and use the equipment at their office or shop.

2. Hire a doctor, nurse practitioner, physician assistant, nurse or tattoo removal technician who already has a business to visit your location on a regular basis. They may be able to bring portable equipment, or you can rent it. We've included a list of laser device rental companies listed on pages 38–40 of this guide that could supply the devices.

3. Look around to see if your area has a mobile tattoo removal clinic. Although these are still rare, we know of several people who are in the process of setting up this type of operation. One already in existence, Ink 180 in Chicago, connects with churches and community groups to do weekly tattoo removal clinics. It owns an RV and two retired ambulances, which it uses to run these clinics at locations around the Chicago area. It has also done them in Detroit, Kansas City and Minneapolis.

4. Rent a laser device that comes with a nurse, doctor or tattoo removal technician or have the rental company source one for you. (There are two types of technicians that laser device rental companies may be able to supply. One is a tattoo removal technician who does the actual procedures and the other is a technician who comes with the machine to set it up, take it down and make sure it operates correctly.)

5. Send clients to an already existing program.

6. Partner with an existing program in a more formalized manner so that the clients of both programs would be seen during the same time periods.

7. Check with the health education, community education or another similar department at your local area hospitals to see if one of them might be interested in partnering on a program with you. Most hospitals have budgets for community outreach and other programs that could partially or fully fund

your program, and they might offer their site as the location for the pop-up clinic. Nurses and other hospital personnel may be interested in volunteering the day of the program. The health education person might be able to get the word out and recruit participants to help with the intake and screening. Dermatology and plastic surgery departments may also be interested in supporting such a program, using their equipment and facilities. Teaching hospitals may be particularly interested in welcoming a program, because performing the procedures can offer educational and training opportunities for residents, fellows and other clinicians.

Here are some of the things you may need to know if you're thinking about a pop-up program:

- It may cost about $300 to $400 per hour to rent a machine with a nurse provided by the rental company to perform the procedures. (These are San Francisco Bay Area prices. They may differ in other areas of the country.) Some practitioners say they average about eight to 10 treatments per hour, but it depends on what type of tattoos are being removed. They could be anything from tiny teardrops, which take just seconds, to full face tattoos, which could take much, much longer.

- Tattoo removal programs are regulated by state laws, so check to see what is required by the medical board and the board of registered nursing in your state. For example, some states require supervision by a doctor, others have less stringent requirements.

- Determine how often you would like to offer the tattoo removal treatments. Most practitioners recommend at least six weeks or more between treatments so that the client's skin can heal.

- Decide how many volunteers will be necessary. Volunteers may be needed to let people into the facility and explain the procedure, for intake (in terms of creating and keeping records), to take before and after photos, if that's something the organization would like to do or any other duties your organization might feel necessary. You may want to contact another program listed in our Tattoo Removal Directory on pages 68–93, with the most current version at www.jailstojobs.org to see just how many people are involved in their process.

Laser device companies and their products

While many companies manufacture laser equipment for a wide variety of medical uses, only about 15 actually produce or sell laser devices that remove tattoos.

This is a list of those companies and details about them and some of their products. Since new products may be released in the future, however, it's best to check out the company websites for their current offerings.

All of these companies are members of the American Society of Laser Medicine and Surgery. You can find out more about the organization at www.aslms.org.

Aerolase Corporation

777 Old Saw Mill River Road
Tarrytown, NY 10591
914-345-8300
www.aerolase.com

Aerolase produces the LightPodNeo, which employs a new 650-microsecond technology able to deliver the same range of laser energy as longer pulsed lasers but with a shorter duration. This results in less heat generation and, the manufacturer says, no discomfort. It is effective in reducing black, blue, green and other dark pigments and complements the Q-switched Nd:YAG and Alexandrite lasers that are traditionally used for tattoo removal. Its ability to produce intense pulses aids in the removal of deep tattoos.

Alma Lasers, Inc.

485 Half Day Road, Suite 100
Buffalo Grove, IL 60089
866-414-2562
224-377-2161
www.almalasers.com

Alma Lasers sells the Harmony Family platform. The platform has 70 different clinical and aesthetic applications, but practitioners only have to buy the ones they need. For tattoo removal, that would be the company's Q-switched Nd:YAG hand piece, which uses two wavelengths to treat a broad range of tattoo colors.

Astanza Laser, Inc.

1770 St. James Place
Houston, TX 77056
800-364-9010
www.astanzalaser.com

Astanza manufacturers three different laser devices. The Astanza Duality Nd:YAG laser, an active Q-switched system which the company calls the workhorse of laser devices, can remove nearly 95% of all tattoo colors. Another Nd:YAG laser, the Astanza Revolution with a passive Q-switch system, at 36 lbs. is portable and easy to use. The Astanza Eternity, an active Q-switched ruby laser, is used to treat colors, like lime green and sky blue that other lasers can't.

Cutera

3240 Bayshore Blvd.
Brisbane, CA 94005
415-657-5500
www.cutera.com

Cutera has launched its enlighten, a laser platform featuring dual wavelength and both picosecond and nanosecond pulse durations which clear a wide range of tattoo colors, ink compositions and pigment concerns.

Cynosure, Inc.

5 Carlisle Road
Westford, MA 01886
978-256-4200
www.cynosure.com

Cynosure produces the PicoSure, a picosecond laser device designed to more effectively treat red, yellow and orange tattoo ink colors, and the RevLite SI, its new generation Q-switched Nd:YAG device that treats multi-color tattoos.

Ellman International, Inc.

400 Karin Lane
Hicksville, NY 11801
800-835-5355
www.ellman.com

Ellman International, a Cynosure company, offers a variety of laser equipment. Its Medley Multifunction Laser Platform provides multiple technologies that include Q-switched Nd:YAG & KTP, Erbium YAG and Intense Pulsed Light. The company also sells the Ruby Q-switched laser that removes multiple and difficult tattoo inks.

Focus Medical

23 Francis J Clarke Circle
Bethel, CT 06801
866-633-5273
www.focusmedical.com

Focus Medical manufacturers the NaturaLase QS Q-switched YAG Laser, originally designed by John Lee, the company's CEO. The machine has four different Q-switched wavelengths and, besides tattoos, can remove unwanted hair, age spots and vascular lesions. The company introduced its PiQo4™ system, the first picosecond laser with four wavelengths in fall 2015. The new device is distributed by Zarin Medical in North America.

Fotona Lasers

1241 Puerta del Sol
San Clemente, CA 92673
949-276-6650
www.fotona.com

Founded in 1964, Ljubljana, Slovenia-headquartered Fotona develops lasers for medical, dental, and industry and defense purposes. The company produces the QX MAX laser system which offers four wavelengths that make it possible to treat almost every pigment color.

Light Age, Inc.

500 Apgar Drive
Somerset, NY 08873
732-563-0600
www.lightage.com

Light Age manufactures a variety of lasers, including the Ta2Eraser, a Q-switched Alexandrite laser which specializes in removing black, blue, brown and green tattoo pigments, as well as various lesions. It can either complement or be used as an alternative to a Q-switched Nd: YAG laser.

Lumenis Aesthetic

2033 Gateway Place, Suite 200
San Jose, CA 95110
408-764-3000
www.lumenis.com

A division of Yokneam, Israel-headquartered Lumenis Ltd., Lumenis Aesthetic sells the Lumenis Q-swtiched Nd:YAG, which employs a top hat beam profile and has the versatility of five spot sizes. It is especially effective for the removal of dark tattoos and is among the safest options for use on people of color.

Lutronic, Inc.

850 Auburn Court
Fremont, CA 94538
888-588-7644
www.usa.lutronic.com

Lutronic manufactures the dual-pulsed Q-switched Nd: YAG SPECTRA laser, which has four wavelengths for a range of treatments, including melisma.

Medicol USA

P.O. Box 186
New Almaden, CA 95042
408-732-6575
www.medicolusa.com

Medicol manufactures and distributes a wide variety of medical equipment, including a Q-switched Nd: YAG laser device.

Perigee Medical

460 W. Larch Road, Suite 25
Tracy, CA 95304
844-737-4433
www.perigeemedical.com

Perigee Medical sells its TattooStar Combo as either a stand-alone system or modular Q-switched multi-wavelength system based on technology developed by Germany's Asclepion Laser Technologies. The TattooStar delivers square beam profiles that the company says offer a 30% improvement in coverage over other methods, without the need to overlap.

Syneron Candela

530 Boston Post Road
Wayland, MA 01778
800-733-8550
www.syneron-candela.com

Although Syneron Candela is one company, it has three brands Syneron, Candela and CoolTouch. Its sells the Picoway, a dual wavelength picosecond laser, as well as the Alex TriVantage Q-switched Alexandrite laser with multi wavelengths. Both are effective for multicolor tattoo removal and an ability to treat a variety of pigmented lesions.

Quanta Aesthetic Lasers

384 Inverness Parkway, Suite 125
Englewood, CO 80112
888-595-2869
www.quantausa.com

Founded in 1985 by an Italian doctor, Quanta Aesthetic Lasers sells a variety of devices that include the Q-Plus series of tattoo removal devices, which offers three laser wavelengths.

Service and repair, parts and used lasers

Many laser device related companies are caring and philanthropic in nature and frequently are open to offering discounts to community-based programs and nonprofits. Remember to always ask about what is available.

Directed Light, Inc.
74 Bonaventura Dr.
San Jose, CA 95134
408-321-8500
www.directedlight.com

Direct Light, Inc. does laser device contract manufacturing and machining, as well as laser components sales and service for medical and industrial clients.

Laser Scientific
210 Commerce Blvd., Suite A
Round Rock, TX, 78664
512-733-8709
www.laserscientific.com

Laser Scientific designs and manufactures laser device replacement parts, components and accessories. It also offers nationwide on-site repair of laser equipment.

TJS, Inc.
4355 Saint Johns Parkway
Sanford, FL 32771
407-328-0777
www.tjslasers.com

TJS, Inc. has been offering laser components, repairs, services and refurbishing for the medical and aesthetic, industrial, scientific and semiconductor markets for more than three decades.

Laser device rental companies

One easy way to launch a program is to rent a machine that comes with a nurse or a technician. Some programs may want to rent a laser device even if they have a doctor or nurse of their own, because it might be cost effective to do so.

Here's a comprehensive list of laser device rental companies, but there may be others. We've found that nonprofit and community-based programs can usually obtain a discount off of their standard rates. Be sure to ask and negotiate.

Aesthetic Laser Partners

11212 Old Georgetown Road
Rockville, MD 20852
301-758-2516
www.aestheticlasersnow.com
Rental delivery area: Maryland

Aesthetic Mobile Laser

905 E. Hillsboro Blvd.
Deerfield Beach, FL 33441
954-522-8477
www.aestheticmobilelaser.com
Rental delivery area: South and Central Florida

ForTec Medical

10125 Wellman Road
Streetsboro, OH 44241
800-963-7101
www.fortecmedical.com
Rental delivery area: National

Laser Service Solutions

200 Grove Road, Suite H
Paulshoro, NJ 08066
856-853-7555
www.Laserservicesolutions.com
Rental delivery area: New Jersey, New York, Pennsylvania and Delaware

Medical Laser Rental and Service Company

4740-A Interstate Drive
Cincinnati, OH 45246
513-489-5595
www.medicallaserrental.com
Rental delivery area: Cincinnati, Ohio

Medical Laser Technologies

1 Walton Road
Seabrook, NH 03874
800-905-5273
www.medlasertech.com
Rental delivery area: Connecticut, Massachusetts, Maine, New Hampshire, New Jersey, New York, Pennsylvania, Rhode Island and Vermont

Monarch Aesthetic Services (Northern California)

25125 Santa Clara St.
Hayward, CA 94544
800-251-2190
www.monarchlasers.com
Rental delivery area: San Francisco Bay Area

Monarch Aesthetic Services (Southern California)

27071 Cabot Road, Suite 113
Laguna Hills, CA 92653
866-599-5570
www.monarchlasers.com
Rental delivery area: Los Angeles and surrounding area; Las Vegas and Southerland, Nev.; and Phoenix and Scottsdale, Ariz.

Southern Medical Lasers

1819 Two Notch Road
Lexington, SC 29073
803-513-8310
www.smlasers.com
Rental delivery area: North Carolina, South Carolina and Georgia

Southland Surgical Laser

2301 E. 28th St., Suite 307
Signal Hill, CA 90755
562-490-4651
www.southlandlaserrental.com
Rental delivery area: Southern California

Texas Laser Source

1730 Jefferson St., Suite 219
Houston, TX 77003
844-995-2737
www.texaslasersource.com
Rental delivery area: Houston and Austin, Texas

UHS Surgical Services

10939 Pendleton St.
Sun Valley, CA 91352
800-660-6162
www.uhssurgicalservices.com
Rental delivery area: National

West Coast Laser

4850 SW Scholls Ferry Road, Suite 109
Portland, OR 97225
503-291-6959
www.westcoastlaser.com
Rental delivery area: Washington and Oregon

Learning the process

Although there are a variety of laser tattoo removal programs at schools around the country, some only offer one-day or two-day courses. We only included the more extensive programs here, with the exception of one school that offers two-day programs around the world. Inclusion, however, doesn't mean we endorse these schools. Potential students have to do their own research to decide if a program is the right one for them.

A Laser Academy

www.alaseracademy.com

Co-founded by well-known tattoo artist Jeff Goyette, this school has three locations: Littleton, Colo., Portsmouth, R.I., and Henderson, Nev. It only teaches tattoo removal—no other procedures—and students work in real-life clinics. The Portsmouth and Henderson locations offer courses every month, but the Rhode Island location—the Inflicting Ink tattoo studio—is just for advanced students who already have two years of experience.

The three–day course is for physicians and their medical staffs, as well as aestheticians and tattoo artists who want to expand what they have to offer. It focuses on hands-on experience rather than just theory. On completing the course, students receive two certifications—Laser Tattoo Removal Specialist and Laser Safety Officer.

National Laser Institute

www.nationallaserinstitute.com

Headquartered in Scottsdale, Ariz., the National Laser Institute has 10 campuses across the country. The campuses are located in San Francisco, New York, Chicago, Newport Beach (L.A. area), Scottsdale, Las Vegas, Seattle, Colorado, Dallas and Philadelphia.

The National Laser Institute offers two-week training courses in a variety of laser and medical aesthetic procedures. There is a core course that covers various procedures and another course that just concentrates on tattoo removal.

In addition, the school offers one-day to three-day continuing education courses for doctors and nurses. At least 15 instructors teach each of the programs, and they include dermatologists, plastic surgeons, aesthetic nurses and others.

New Look Laser College

www.newlooklasercollege.com

Located in Houston, New Look Laser College is the training facility for Astanza Laser, a medical device manufacturer. Its two-day course on tattoo removal is taught around the world in countries including New Zealand, China, England and Denmark. The trainers have operated a tattoo removal clinic, and the emphasis is on practical applications.

Students gain experience in a clinic setting, where patients are treated for free. The curriculum includes the physics of lasers, the treatment of patients, laser safety training, and business operations and marketing. In the U.S., training is conducted six times per year at the Texas facility.

Rocky Mountain Laser College

www.rockymountainlasercollege.com

The Rocky Mountain Laser College offers the Certified Laser Specialist training program, which includes a 20-hour online course and a seven-unit 40-hour on-site training course at the college's Denver-area campus. Those who complete the course receive a Certified Laser Specialist credential.

Professional associations

These associations could be useful for recruiting medical professionals and keeping abreast of changes in technology and best practices in the science of tattoo removal. They may also have local chapters or societies in your area. In addition, your local county medial society and state medical association could also be good recources.

American Society of Cosmetic Physicians

www.cosmeticphysicians.org
520-574-1050

The goal of the Tucson, Ariz.-based American Society of Cosmetic Physicians is to educate physicians, regardless of specialty, on cosmetic procedures through workshops conducted around the U.S. and an annual conference.

American Academy of Dermatology

www.aad.org
866-503-7546

Based in Schaumburg, Ill., and founded in 1938, the American Academy of Dermatology is the main organization for dermatologists and has a membership of more than 17,000 members representing dermatologists both in the U.S. and abroad.

American Society of Dermatologic Surgery

www.asds.net
847-956-0900

Headquartered in Rolling Meadows, Ill, the American Society of Dermatologic Surgery has more than 5,800 members.

American Society for Laser Medicine and Surgery

www.aslms.org
715-845-9283

Headquartered in Wausau, Wis., the American Society for Laser Medicine and Surgery's 3,500 members —15% of whom are outside the U.S.—represent physicians, surgeons, nurses and other healthcare professionals, as well as scientists and engineers involved with product development and laser device manufacturers.

American Society of Plastic Surgeons

www.plasticsurgery.org
847-228-9900

With headquarters in Arlington Heights, Ill., and offices in Dallas and Washington, D.C., the American Society of Plastic Surgeons was founded in 1931 and has 7,000 physician members.

North American Association for Light Therapy

www.naalt.org

The Coeymans Hollow, N.Y.-based North American Association for Light Therapy is an association for therapeutic light therapy practitioners in the U.S., Canada and Mexico.

Optical Society of America

www.osa.org
202-223-8130

Founded in 1916, the Optical Society of America, headquartered in Washington, D.C., with local sections in North America, Asia and Europe, is made up of a membership of science, engineering and business professionals who deal in the fields of optics and photonics. Many physicians who use lasers in their practices are also members.

PanAmerican Photodynamic Association

www.papdt.org

This Minneapolis, Minn.-based association is dedicated to educating scientists, healthcare professionals and the public in the Americas in order to promote the practice of photodynamic therapy techniques.

SPIE (The International Society for Optics and Photonics)

www.spie.org
360-676-3290

With approximately 18,000 members around the globe, the Bellingham, Wash.-headquartered SPIE is dedicated to advancing emerging light-based technologies through, among other things, its many technical forums, exhibitions and educational programs in North America, Asia, Europe and Australia each year.

Tennessee Society for Laser Medicine and Surgery

www.tnlasersociety.com
615-460-1650

The Tennessee Society for Laser Medicine and Surgery, based in Nashville, Tenn., is a membership organization composed of physicians, nurses, engineers, scientists, technologists and other healthcare professionals who deal with laser technology.

Potential funders

The IRS requires nonprofit hospitals to allocate a portion of their budget to improve the health of the communities in which they serve. Fulfilling these community benefit requirements could come in the form of grants, sponsorships, in-kind donations, and charitable contributions. Community health improvement involving prevention such as a community-based tattoo removal program might be an ideal way for hospitals to fulfill this government requirement.

The Second Chance Act supports work to reduce recidivism and improve outcomes for those in reentry. The U.S. Department of Justice's Office of Justice Programs (OJP) funds and administers the Second Chance Act grants. For more details see www.csgjusticecenter.org/nrrc/projects/second-chance-act.

Astanza Laser, Inc. has created a program called Astanza Giving Back. Since 2007 it has been offering free services in the Houston area, where it is located, and since 2009 has provided discounts on its top-of-the-line laser systems to a number of qualified nonprofits and governmental agencies in this field.

Many other programs have received free or discounted tattoo removal training courses conducted by its staff. The company has also made in-kind donations of staff time performing or supervising laser tattoo removal procedures.

ForTec Medical, a laser device rental company in Streetsboro, Ohio, has donated equipment to programs.

Local service clubs like Rotary, Kiwanis, Lions, Optimists, Soroptimists and HandsOn Network are potential funders. They might be willing to sponsor individuals who want to get their tattoos removed or donate toward the purchase of a tattoo laser device.

Government funding is another possibility. In California, for example, CalGRIP (California Gang Reduction, Intervention and Prevention) has given money to tattoo removal programs.

Inmate welfare funds also might be a potential funding source for programs that want to include pre-release inmates.

Another avenue to explore is soliciting donations online through crowdsourcing sites. Gofundme, Kickstarter, Indiegogo, and Crowdfunder are the most popular of these websites, and there are others that might be worth considering too.

Many laser device companies are caring and philanthropic in nature and frequently are open to offering significant discounts to community-based programs and nonprofits. Remember to always ask about what is available.

Possible partners and resources

Those thinking about setting up a free or low-cost program may not want to—or be able to—do it alone. In some cases, having another community partner would be the way to go, and even if someone sets up a clinic on their own, they still might need to establish partnerships to get client referrals.

Here are potential partners to work with. There may be other possibilities, but this is a start:

- A local sheriff's department gang unit (More than 300 of the nation's large police departments also have these gang units)
- Police departments or police auxiliaries
- Gang task forces
- Sheriff's departments without gang units
- Gang intervention organizations and programs
- US Department of Justice, Office of Justice Programs, Office of Juvenile Justice and Delinquency Prevention
- Parole departments
- Probation departments
- FBI (for those dealing with victims of human trafficking)
- Homeland Security (also for those dealing with victims of human trafficking)
- Federal Gang Reduction Intervention Program (GRIP)
- Crimesolutions.gov
- Nationalgangcenter.gov
- Nonprofit organizations
- Faith-based organizations
- Boys & Girls Clubs
- Military recruiters
- County Youth Authority programs
- Community Action Partnership
- City governments
- Employment training organizations that deal with formerly gang-involved and/or previously incarcerated men and women
- Nonprofit hospitals and their Community Benefit resources

Tips and advice from those who've done it

Santa Paula Tattoo Removal Program
Santa Paula, Calif.

- Have conversations with elected officials about the benefits of removing tattoos. For every dollar invested in their county for tattoo removal (supplies, etc.), it received $25 in return just in community service.
- The big expense is the laser. If you have a physician who buys the laser they can use it in their practice for cosmetic treatments.
- Get funding from the local police department or parole office. There's a lot of facial tattooing going on in prison, so they're interested.
- Get a location right where your clients are. We are using a county clinic for indigent patients.
- You need a good point person for the volunteer work.
- Be consistently available.

Second Chance Grace
Meridian, Idaho

- Check local and state requirements ahead of time, since every state has different laws governing tattoo removal and who can do it.
- Find a clinic, existing program or medical facility to partner with. It's easier that way.

Removing Barriers
San Pablo, Calif.

- Talk to employers that may have employees in the back office who have tattoos but want to move to a public area. Get employees of those companies to volunteer. They're professional.
- Have a locked file cabinet for records to ensure HIPPA privacy.
- You need a really good camera that has a macro function to take before-and-after pictures.
- Set up a place in the waiting room where a same sex person can take a photo of all the tattoos.
- Make sure your forms are translated. Fifty percent of those we serve are Latinos.
- Create a set of rules regarding safety.

The former Agape Light Tattoo Removal Program
Culver City Seventh Day Adventist Church
Culver City, Calif.

- Be very open minded and accepting of people who are not going to look like your church members but often have a bigger heart than some of your church members do.
- Look for funding. It might not be fair to have the doctor totally responsible for that. It needs to be a coordinated effort.

Fairfax Skin Deep Tattoo Removal Program
Fairfax, Va.

- Have plenty of space, including a secure registration area, since anyone can walk in off the street; a room for pre-treatment interviews and photos; a treatment room; and a post-treatment room.
- Create a procedure manual with rules and regulations.
- Make sure you get a laser that removes the colors you desire, since not all lasers remove all colors.
- Carefully consider the pros and potential cons of the agency you plan to partner with.
- Have enough money upfront to pay for anesthetic drugs and post-op dressing and medication.

Taboo Tattoo Removal Program
Napa, Calif.

- Because counties want to help local youth and keep their communities free from gangs, get the local county officials involved and talk to them about the importance of helping divert at-risk youth from gangs.

D-Tag Tattoo Removal Program
Carrollton, Texas

- Look into hospitals that will donate space. They are a safe environment, and you have access to services and equipment, in the case of an emergency.
- Always remember that tattoo removal is a medical procedure, and you need a medical record for each and every client.
- Make sure you have liability insurance.
- Use prior programs and success stories from other tattoo clinics to sell your idea.
- If your program is a nonprofit it should be audited every two years in order to be able to apply for grants. 990's and tax returns are very important.
- Always have a medical director on-hand at your clinic, in case there's a problem, and also because they have liability insurance, so you won't be sued.
- Recruit a physician to volunteer.

Homeboy Industries
Los Angeles, Calif.

- Always hire from your own community. People from your own community will work harder and want to make a difference.

Protecting the liability of clinicians and programs

While liability may be a concern to organizations and those thinking about volunteering for or creating a tattoo removal program, none of the doctors or programs we've talked to—and some have been in existence for 15 or 20 years—have ever been sued. In fact, they said that people were very appreciative of the service they provided in removing their tattoos. Our survey covered a variety of programs and sizes, including a single program that served over 3,000 men and women and removed 43,000 tattoos last year alone, with procedures performed by 35 volunteer physicians.

If doctors are performing the removals, they should already have malpractice insurance (a type of professional liability insurance) in place for their own practices which should cover them for their related volunteer work.

The programs themselves, tattoo removal technicians and those needing liability insurance can obtain a professional liability insurance policy from an insurance company, of which there are many to choose from. One such organization is the Professional Program Insurance Brokerage (PPIB) (www.ppibcorp.com) that specializes in covering a wide range of individuals and establishments like medispas, medical laboratories and clinics and those who use lasers for procedures.

Programs can also add doctors and other healthcare professionals to the policies they purchase. A policy from PPIB may be purchased through any commercial insurance broker or directly from PPIB itself. It is also a good idea to consult with your insurance professional for their ideas and suggestions.

There is additional liability protection for volunteers themselves in every state but New Hampshire under the Federal Volunteer Protection Act. Some states also have laws that provide protection for volunteers. Although this act does not replace the need to maintain insurance for programs and volunteers, depending on the state, it can provide additional significant protection for the people who perform any service on a volunteer basis. However, it's important to check out the law in your state to see exactly what it covers.

In addition, there are measures that must be taken beyond making sure that your equipment is functioning and the people performing the procedures are competent at what they do.

The most important of these is to have all patients sign a release form. With one exception, everyone we talked to uses the same form, but they sometimes customize it to fit their own situation. This form can be found on the website of the Professional Program Insurance Brokerage at www.ppibcorp.com/client-forms.html and may be used free of charge.

Case studies

Agape Light Tattoo Removal Program

Culver City Seventh Day Adventist Church
11828 W. Washington Blvd.
Los Angeles, CA 90066
Contact: Pastor Jan Kaatz
310-398-9205
www.culvercity.adventistfaith.org

Although the Agape Light Tattoo Removal Program is currently on hiatus, it may be the only tattoo removal program in the country that was ever actually operated by a church. And for that reason it is included here.

Agape Light was created by a Seventh Day Adventist doctor at a small church in San Pedro, a Los Angeles suburb bordering the ports of Los Angeles and Long Beach. It later moved to the Seventh Day Adventist Church in Burbank, where it operated for eight years and then to a sister church in Culver City, where it ran for another five years until an illness by the pastor put the program on hold a couple of years ago.

How it worked

Those who wanted their tattoos removed were required to come to a Friday night worship service where they would get a voucher for the next treatment date, which was two months later. The doctor removed tattoos from 4 p.m. to 6 p.m. on selected Friday nights throughout the year. He would do exposed—neck up and wrist down—tattoos for free and any others for low-cost. About 35 people had tattoo removal treatments during each of the clinic sessions.

While people were waiting for their treatments, Pastor Kaatz would talk to them to find out what was going on in their lives and pray with them, if they were open to that idea. Afterwards they would all go together for a meal at the church and then the Friday evening service, where they would get vouchers for their next treatment.

Besides church attendance, 10 hours of community service was required between treatments. According to Pastor Kaatz, the community service was defined loosely as helping someone besides themselves and did not have to be in connection with an official organization. It could also be for volunteering in their local church with youth groups or whatever.

The equipment

The laser was the property of the volunteer doctor, and part of the reason the church decided to end the program was because the laser was getting worn out and there was no funding to replace it.

D-Tag Tattoo Removal Program

4325 N. Josey Lane #107
Carrollton, TX 75010
Contact: Cia Bond, *Executive Director, Metrocrest Medical Foundation*
cbond@mmftx.org
972-247-0286
www.mmftx.org

D-Tag is one of the programs of the Metrocrest Medical Foundation (MMF), the fundraising arm of the Metrocrest Hospital Authority (MHA).

Created in 1995 by local dermatologist Dr. Dennis Newton, D-Tag is geared to young people leaving the gang life or individuals who want to join the military. The program is now a partnership between the following organizations and people, who all volunteer their time:

- Three dermatologists (Dr. Mike Maris, Dr. Rebecca Euwer and Dr. Newton) do the procedures.
- M. Wallace, a laser technician, assists the doctors and provides laser machine training.
- MMF D-Tag Tattoo Removal Program is a training site for the dermatology residents of UT Southwest Medical School Dallas.
- School nurses from the Carrollton-Farmers Branch Independent School District assist doctors and handle appointments.
- Dermatology Consultants donates the space where the procedures are performed.
- The Carrollton/Farmers Branch Police Department recommends students and appears at each session.

How it works

The program removes homemade gang tattoos and tattoos restricted by the military that are visible on the hands, arms, neck or face.

The youth clients are referred by local schools and police departments, as well as the courts. In order to enter the program they must apply with an application form and two letters of recommendation—one from a mentor who helps them with their community service requirement and the other from a parent, teacher or minister. If under 18 years of age, their parent or guardian is required to attend the first treatment session. Clients must perform 10 hours of community service before each treatment.

Six sessions per year are conducted in donated space within the hospital. The facilities include a day surgery unit and two outpatient surgery spaces.

The procedure/equipment

The doctors had been using rather old laser equipment donated by a laser technician to perform the equivalent of $135,000 worth of treatments per year. In March 2014 Metrocrest Medical Foundation raised $40,000 to purchase a new-used Candela Laser Machine.

Although all the personnel volunteer their time, there are expenses such as medical supplies and equipment repair that are covered by the Metrocrest Medical Foundation, which D-Tag operates under the auspices of.

Fairfax Skin Deep Tattoo Removal Program

Fairfax County Health Department
Fairfax, VA
703-246-8751
www.fairfaxcounty.gov/hd/tattoo

A partnership between the cities of Fairfax and Falls Church, Va., Fairfax County public service agencies and nonprofit organizations, the Fairfax Skin Deep Program was created in 1997 as a way to get young people out of gangs. The focus is on youth aged 14 to 22.

Although the stated purpose is to remove tattoos, the ultimate goals include to reduce crime, improve educational opportunities, provide alternatives to gangs, provide community service opportunities and ultimately to develop employed tax-paying citizens.

How it works

There are only about 10 young people enrolled in the program at a time, because the procedures are done after hours, when plastic surgeon doctors and nurses, who are on the county government payroll, are available to remove tattoos. Representatives from county human service agencies volunteer their time to run the office and do the behind-the-scenes work.

The youth are required to put in 40 community service hours before their tattoos will be removed for free and are monitored for drug and alcohol use. Drug tests are administered, and if either is suspected of being used, participants will be thrown out of the program immediately.

The equipment

They rent a YAG laser device paid for with funds from Fairfax County.

City of Fresno Mayor's Gang Prevention Initiative

2323 Mariposa St.
Fresno, CA 93721
Contact: Maggie Navarro, *Communications Coordinator*
Maggie.navarro@fresno.gov
559-621-6213
www.fresno.gov/Government/DepartmentDirectory/Police/AboutFresnoPD/
PoliceServicesandSpecialUnits/MayorsGangPreventionInitiative.htm

The City of Fresno, Calif., has been running a tattoo removal clinic for more than five years as part of the Mayor's Gang Prevention Initiative (MGPI), which works to reduce the number of gang-related crimes in Fresno.

The process incorporates five core components: prevention, intervention, suppression, rehabilitation and economic development and removal of gang tattoos falls under the intervention component.

The police department has negotiated an agreement with the Fresno County Economic Opportunities Commission (FCEOC) for tattoo removal services. Under the most recent Memorandum of Understanding, which covers the period from June 1, 2012 to Dec. 31, 2014, the city reimbursed the FCEOC for up to $50,000, with the money coming from grant funds.

How it works

FCEOC provides part-time clinic facilities and a medical staff—a doctor and nurse practitioner—who conduct a weekly clinic every Tuesday. They remove tattoos from people referred by the Mayor's Gang Prevention Initiative.

Those who get their tattoo removed are not charged for the treatments but must be enrolled in the Mayor's Gang Prevention Initiative. The program first does a needs assessment of potential participants. Once people are determined appropriate for the program, they are assigned a case manager, who facilitates treatment services depending on need.

Besides tattoo removal, these include mental and substance abuse treatment, help with anger management, assistance with education (GED, higher education, tutoring), and job training and placement. Depending on the availability of funding, there might also be help with housing and transportation.

Other requirements:

- Must be a resident of the city of Fresno.
- Must have a direct gang affiliation.
- Must not have a pending case, warrant or other disqualifying conviction.
- Must perform at least 20 community service hours per month at an approved location for the duration of the treatment period, which averages five to 10 months.
- Sex offenders are not allowed into the program.

The procedure/equipment

The clinic uses a Medlite C6 Q-switched laser that was purchased by the Fresno Police Department with CalGRIP (California Gang Reduction, Intervention and Prevention) funds when the program began. CalGRIP is a statewide funding program launched in 2007 by Governor Arnold Schwarzenegger to help address the increasing presence of gangs across the state.

Homeboy Industries

130 West Bruno St.
Los Angeles, CA 90012
Contact: Esmeralda Mendez, *Tattoo Removal Manager*
emendez@homeboyindustries.org
323-526-1254, x344
www.homeboyindustries.org

Homeboy Industries operates the biggest free tattoo removal clinic in the country. It is one of the many programs run by the 27-year old organization that was founded by Father Greg Boyle and offers an array of free services to formerly gang-involved and previously incarcerated men and women.

Many clients are referred by probation officers and schools, and the clinic also works with half a dozen or so juvenile facilities, bringing the inmates to the clinic to have their tattoos removed so that they're ready to search for employment upon release.

Homeboy Industries has found that tattoo removal is often a "gateway service" which leads clients to take further advantage of the organization's other services and programs. These include mental health or substance abuse treatment, skills training and job development.

The organization also believes that removing tattoos will make parents better role models.

How it works

Although very small in size, with only two 8' x 11' treatment rooms and a small waiting area, the clinic serves as many as 950 clients and performs an average of 3,000 tattoo treatments each month. It started with a staff of three but now has a staff of eight, with only one of them, a physician's assistant, who is paid.

Two people work on checking clients in, several handle email and walk-ins—there are about 120 walk-ins per month—and there's a translator. Volunteers work four phones scheduling appointments. Thirty-five doctors volunteer their time to do the removals at various times of the year.

The clinic only removes gang-related tattoos. No one is charged and no community service is required.

The procedure/equipment

The clinic has four Q-switched YAG lasers. In late 2014 Homeboy launched a campaign to raise money to upgrade its tattoo removal laser equipment. Astanza Laser matched the first $100,000 Homeboy raised. One of their four machines is an Astanza and they are in the process of aquiring a second Astanza.

Houston Laser Institute

515 N. Sam Houston Parkway East, Suite 310
Houston, TX 77060
Contact: Wayne Heintze, *Co-Founder*
kingwoodite@yahoo.com
281-789-8636

Houston Laser Institute is a rather new venture, created in January 2013 by Wayne Heintze, the former chaplain and current director of reentry services for Houston's Harris County Sheriff's Department, and his wife, Francine. Inspired by a prisoner who wanted to get his tattoos removed, Heintze took training at a laser college, bought a laser and found a place with month-to-month rent.

Heintze has been operating the Houston Laser Institute for nearly three years and has supported it partially with his own money. He's in the process of creating a nonprofit, however, and intends to eventually offer all of his services free of charge.

How it works

Although Houston Laser Institute has a doctor who acts as medical director as required by Texas law, Heintze does all the procedures himself. He schedules appointments Monday through Friday from 11 a.m. to 7 p.m. and Saturdays from 9 a.m. to 1 p.m., but mostly does them from 3 p.m. to 7 p.m. on weekdays in order to be able to work them into the schedule for his regular job with the sheriff's department.

Heintze, his wife and the doctor all volunteer their time. He gets clients through the Internet and word of mouth and also speaks to a lot of groups because of his work with the reentry program and can publicize the tattoo removal program that way.

The clinic is located in an office building and has three small rooms—a reception area, his own office and a treatment room.

About 90% of Houston Laser Institute's clients consists of previously incarcerated men and women, and the other 10% is made up of police, military and fire personnel. There are no age restrictions, but under-aged youth need parental/guardian permission.

What is charged

The cost per visit for previously incarcerated men and women is $49 plus four hours of community service. The community service must be performed before each visit and verified. He charges others a higher rate but gives military and first responders a 50% discount off of that rate.

Between the rent and other expenses, the program costs about $2,000 per month to operate. The fee Heintze charges covers most of his costs, but he still has to subsidize some of them with his own funds.

The procedure/equipment

Heintze uses a Cynosure C-4 Medlite laser machine that he purchased for $80,000 of his own money to start the program. Appointments are scheduled eight weeks apart.

Ink 180 Mobile Tattoo Removal Program

27 Stonehill Road, Unit D
Oswego, IL 60543
Contact: Chris Baker, *Chief Ink Officer*
chris@ink180.com
630-554-1404
http://ink180.com

Chris Baker, who operates a tattoo shop, and a nonprofit organization that does free tattoo removals and cover-ups—in which a beautiful tattoo is imposed on top of already existing ink—created a mobile operation in spring 2014. Both his nonprofit and mobile unit offer its services free of charge to former gang members, previously incarcerated men and women, victims of sex trafficking and victims of domestic violence.

A Christian, Baker looks at the mobile operation as an extension of the street ministry he does in Chicago. He and a group of volunteers go throughout the inner city of Chicago on a weekly basis and have also visited Detroit, Kansas City and Indianapolis.

How it works

A church, a ministry or other group will approach Ink 180 saying they have a number of people who want gang and other tattoos removed. Baker works with the churches to make it an event that may include various other organizations and providers offering services like GED preparation or dental care.

Tattoo removal appointments are made ahead of time, and he has two or three people ready to volunteer. Baker and his team can perform up to 20 removals per vehicle and have done a total of up to 60 removals in one day.

The procedure/equipment

Baker was able to begin the mobile operation because someone donated an RV to his organization. Word got around, and soon two more vehicles—retired ambulances—were donated. He removes tattoos using intense pulsed light therapy (IPL) rather than a laser device.

Santa Paula Tattoo Removal Program

1334 E. Main St.
Santa Paula, CA 93060
Contact: Martin Hernandez, *Clinic Coordinator*
martin.hernandez@ventura.org
805-933-1242
www.vchca.org

Launched in Santa Paula 15 years ago, the Santa Paula Tattoo Removal Program initially was strictly for parolees and people who were on probation. Its goal was to help gang members get their tattoos removed, and some of the tattoo removals were ordered by a judge. A second clinic was established four years ago in Oxnard. (The two clinics operate almost identically, but with slight differences. This case study focuses on Oxnard.)

Today clients include not only parolees and those on probation but youth from juvenile hall and anyone who wants to get their gang or other tattoos—including exes (ex-girlfriend and boyfriend)—removed but can't afford it. There are no age restrictions. The youngest patient was a four-year-old whose parents tattooed him, and the oldest in his 70s.

How it works
The first treatment is free, but the second requires 40 hours of community service. After the community service is completed, clients can come to the clinic as many times as it takes to have their tattoos removed.

The clinic operates from 8 a.m. to 1 p.m. on the third Saturday of each month, and about 35 people have tattoo removal treatments during each session.

Everyone who works at the clinic volunteers their time, with the exception of one staff member, a receptionist, who is paid by Las Islas Clinic, which donates the space and the numbing cream, dressing and tape.

Five or more volunteers work each clinic session—one or two doctors, a person to do intake, another who does orientation for first-timers, still another who takes a photo before and after the first treatment, and someone to put on topical ointment and explain how to care for the skin where the tattoo has been removed. There's also a volunteer in charge of advising patients on community service options and keeping charts for each person, the treatments they've received and the community service they've performed.

The program is publicized by a free announcement in the local community newspaper that runs one to two weeks before each clinic session. A volunteer recently created a public service announcement, which is running on a local radio station.

The procedure/equipment
The laser equipment was purchased by the Oxnard Police Department through a CalGRIP (Gang Reduction Intervention Program) grant. One of its two lenses is wearing out, and the City of Oxnard has a block grant it planned to use to replace that lens at a cost of about $500.

Removing Barriers
San Pablo Economic Development Corporation
13830 San Pablo Ave., Suite D
San Pablo, CA 94806
Contact: Leslay Choy, *Executive Director*
510-215-3200
www.sanpabloedc.org

The San Pablo Economic Development Corp., in partnership with the City of San Pablo and the San Jose, Calif.-based nonprofit New Skin Adult Tattoo Removal, launched the Removing Barriers program in April 2013.

Although a job training and job readiness program, Removing Barriers includes removal of visible tattoos that could serve as a barrier to employability, safety and reentry. This small San Francisco Bay Area suburb with a population of roughly 29,000 has big intentions to help create a safer more sustainable community with greater opportunities for all.

How it works

The tattoo removal clinic takes place from 8 a.m. to 12 noon on the third Saturday of the month. Appointments are encouraged, but walk-ins are accepted between 9 a.m. and 11 a.m.

According to Leslay Choy, executive director, "the program is open to anybody anywhere, for any reason, and for visible and nonvisible tattoos. It's more about confidence and leaving a past life. We're helping people be confident in the skin they're in and removing barriers to employment and community safety."

Once someone has made an appointment, they will receive an email blast, a personal email and then a phone call, reminding them of their appointment time, how early they have to come, etc. This attention to detail has reduced the no-show rate. Out of 58 to 70 appointments made for each clinic, about 38 to 50 people will show up. In addition, there's an average of six walk-ins.

There are eight staffers, including a paid administrative intern. Volunteers come from the Office of the City of San Pablo, individual volunteers, local companies, local colleges and the local Rotary Club, which also sponsors some of the patients who can't afford the fee.

A police officer always stops by sometime during the morning. "We want people to see their presence and understand our relationship with them," Choy says. "A lot of the police actually have tattoos, so they understand. It's a different connection."

What is charged

There is a charge of $50 per session for San Pablo residents and $75 for non-residents. Those who get tattoos removed may participate in the 10-week job readiness program for free. Those who attend the job readiness program will be reimbursed for their $50 tattoo removal program enrollment fee, and if they complete the program will get two free tattoo removal sessions.

The procedure/equipment

The tattoo removal procedure is performed by a nurse supplied by New Skin Adult Tattoo Removal, a nonprofit organization, who comes with a laser device and sets up the clinic in the San Pablo Economic Development Corporation's office.

Second Chance Grace

P.O. Box 1058
Meridian, ID 83680
Contact: Jeri Vasquez, *Program Manager*
jeri@2ndchancegrace.org
208-703-6930
www.2ndchancegrace.org

Second Chance Grace, a Meridian, Idaho, nonprofit organization dedicated to helping at-risk youth and young adults, decided that one of the ways it could benefit them was by offering to take off their unwanted tattoos.

It teamed up with Eagle River Medical Aesthetics in Boise, about 10 miles away, to create the state's first gang tattoo removal center, which handles about 20 patients per month.

How it works
Clients are first referred to 2nd Chance Grace through probation and parole officers, and drug and alcohol treatment centers. They must participate in a phone screening conducted by Executive Director Peter Vasquez, formerly gang-involved and previously incarcerated himself, who determines their attitude and motivation for removing the tattoo(s).

If people pass the initial screening, the tattoo removal manager calls them and does another phone interview. They then undergo a background check, and if that is satisfactory, fill out an application form. The client is then given a list of community organizations and must pick one of them to volunteer with, which is one of the program's requirements.

All clients must have been out of jail or prison for at least 60 days and have no active warrants. They must also be a U.S. citizen or have a green card. Everyone must be gang-free and working, going to school and/ or enrolled in a vocational or job readiness program.

If they don't show up or call back two times, they can no longer participate.

What is charged
Adults are charged $45 per-tattoo per treatment, but tattoos can't be bigger than their hand. Of that amount, $25 goes to the clinic and $20 to Second Chance Grace's youth fund. Youth under 18 years of age are charged $20 per tattoo per treatment or treated for free if they can't afford the fee. Adults and youth who pay are required to perform 20 hours of community service. Those who obtain free treatments must do 25 hours of community service, with five hours before they receive the first treatment.

The procedure/equipment
All tattoo removal procedures at the Eagle River Medical Aesthetics clinic are performed by a board certified family nurse practitioner or an R.N. The clinic uses the Cynosure's RevLite SI, a new generation Q-switched Nd:YAG that treats multi-color tattoos. The clinic says it was the first facility in the Northwest and the only facility in Idaho to have this laser.

Taboo Tattoo Removal Program
2310 First St.
Napa, CA 94559
Contact: Anna Hernandez, *Program Director*
707-255-1855
www.aldeainc.org

In 1998 a local plastic surgeon saw the need for a tattoo removal program geared toward former youth gang members, and although it initially only accepted youth, adults were soon included as well. Taboo Tattoo now operates as part of Aldea Children & Family Services at Wolfe Center, a substance prevention and treatment program for teenagers.

The clinic takes place one morning a month on either the fourth Tuesday or fourth Thursday, from 7:15 a.m. to 9:00 a.m. Participants are seen on a first-come, first-served basis.

How it works

When the program began more than 15 years ago, the procedures took place in space donated by the Queen of the Valley Medical Center, a Catholic nonprofit hospital. Taboo Tattoo moved to the Napa County Health Department where it operated for a while, but the clinic now takes place in the group room at the Wolfe Center building not far from downtown Napa.

Two doctors do the procedures—one each month—and an Aldea Children & Family Services staff member handles the intake process.

People, who get tattoos removed, with a few exceptions, must be residents of Napa County. Only visible tattoos are removed.

What is charged

There are three conditions under which people can get their tattoos removed:

- Napa County residents between the ages of 13 and 25 currently enrolled in an Alcohol, Drug and Gang-free program (juvenile and adult probation programs) who do not have any new tattoos will receive free tattoo removal treatments. Youth must be enrolled in school and those under age 18 must be accompanied by a parent or probation officer.
- Napa County youth and adults who perform four hours of community service for each treatment session will also get their tattoos removed for free.
- All other participants are expected to contribute a suggested donation of $50 per treatment.

The procedure/equipment

Taboo Tattoo rents the laser equipment, which comes with a technician. Although it costs $900 per month, Queen of the Valley Medical Center pays for the rental, as well as various ointments and other medical supplies.

Pre-release tattoo removal programs

Why should people wait until after getting out of jail or prison to get tattoos removed? And why don't more places have pre-release tattoo removal programs?

Those that don't may want to follow the lead of the Los Angeles Sheriff's Department, Kern County (Calif.) Probation Department, the Oregon Youth Authority and Travis County (Texas) Jail, all of which have tattoo removal programs for inmates. There may be others, but these are the ones we are most familiar with, and here's the rundown.

Los Angeles County Sheriff's Department Tattoo Removal Program
450 Bauchet St., Room E873
Los Angeles, CA 90012
213-893-5445
www.lasd.org

A collaborative partnership between The Los Angeles County Sheriff's Department Medical Services Bureau and the Inmate Services Bureau, the L.A. County Sheriff's Tattoo Removal Program has treated more than 500 inmates since it was launched in early 2012 with 25 volunteer inmates.

The tattoo removal program is overseen by trained medical personnel and paid for with money from the Inmate Welfare Fund. The focus is on gang-affiliation tattoos or tattoos that will prohibit those who have them from gaining employment.

Tattoo removal sessions take place every Tuesday and Thursday from 2:30 p.m. to 8:30 p.m. at Twin Towers Correctional Facility and North County Correctional Facility. The procedures are performed by L.A. Sheriff Department nurses who have been trained by a doctor from the laser device company.

In order to take advantage of the program, inmates must either be a jail trustee with a low security level or participate in the LASD's Education-Based Incarceration program, through which they can obtain diplomas, GEDs, vocational certificates for various trades and even college degrees during the time that they're incarcerated. Getting tattoos removed is considered a sort of reward for their hard work and will result in a better outcome for the inmates once released.

"Visible tattoos, especially those that are gang-related or profane, can negatively impact an inmate's ability to find employment after their release. An ex-inmate who can find a job is better able to reintegrate into the community, and less likely to end up back in jail," says Medical Services Bureau Captain Kevin Kuykendall. "This program helps those inmates that have made the commitment to better themselves while in custody carry that commitment with them as they re-enter our communities."

Kern County, Calif. Take Away Tattoos Program

2005 Ridge Road
Bakersfield, CA 93305
Contact: Elaine Moore, *Supervisor*
elainemoore@co.kern.ca.us
661-868-4519
http://kernprobation.com/pack/

This program is operated by P.A.C.K., the Probation Auxiliary County of Kern, a nonprofit arm of the Kern County, Calif., probation department. Kern County includes the city of Bakersfield. The program began in 1998 and for most of its history has concentrated on juveniles in custody and on probation. Things changed once AB109—the California Assembly Bill that allows individuals sentenced to non-serious, non-violent or non-sex offences to serve their sentences in county jails instead of state prisons—got into full swing. Now the program treats people on probation and those under AB109, who can begin treatments while in custody and finish post-release.

The Take Away Tattoos program had been just for those on probation, but beginning in January 2014 it was opened to inmates.

The procedures take place twice monthly in clinic space donated by a local nonprofit health agency, Clinica Sierra Vista. They are performed by four volunteer physician assistants—a different one each week—overseen by a doctor who has been with the program since the beginning.

Those getting their tattoos removed are from the Kern County Jail and referred by jail staff based on their performance in the programs they're participating in while in custody.

Previously, adults were charged $50 per session and juveniles were required to do community service, but those requirements were dropped, because they were able to buy new laser tattoo removal devices with AB 109 funds.

Medical supplies are provided by Clinica Sierra Vista, and nursing students from a local junior college are brought to each clinic session with their teachers to do pre- and post-treatment bandaging and give post-treatment instructions.

Oregon Youth Authority's Tattoo Removal Program

Office of Inclusion and Intercultural Relations
Oregon Youth Authority
530 Center St. NE, Suite 200
Salem, OR 97301
503-378-4667
http://www.oregon.gov/oya/pages/oms.aspx

Coordinated by the state's Office of Inclusion and Intercultural Relations, the Oregon Youth Authority's Tattoo Removal Program was founded by a group of psychiatrists who thought that it would be important for young people to get rid of their gang tattoos. In recent years it has been run by Carolyn Hale, a volunteer dermatologist, who was joined in late 2014 by four local retired doctors, a nurse and a physician's assistant.

Hale is a strong believer in volunteerism and thinks what she's doing is especially important. "They're (the kids) are not really educated as to what it means when they get their gang tattoos. To get out of the gang life they have to get rid of those gang tattoos. It's dangerous for them to leave the youth facility with gang tattoos," she says.

Although they currently perform tattoo removals once a month at the state's main facility for juvenile offenders, the Oregon Youth Facility at the Hillcrest Youth Correctional Facility, which has a medical clinic, they hope to be able to soon increase that to at least three times per month. The kids come from a variety of places – the boys from four facilities and the girls from one.

The multicultural coordinator of the Oregon Youth Authority's Office of Inclusion and Intercultural Relations also serves as coordinator of the tattoo removal program. Once the kids have been in the program, they can come back and receive more tattoo removal treatments, even after they are released from the youth authority facility.

The youth who participate cannot have any discipline problems and need to be making a sincere effort to get out of a gang. They also have to commit to having all of their gang tattoos removed.

Although the doctors who originally started the program bought the first laser device with grant money, when that device broke and needed to be replaced, one of the original doctors and Dr. Hale bought the next one with their own money, helped by a significant discount given by the laser device manufacturer.

Travis County (Texas) Jail Pre-release Tattoo Removal Program

500 W 10th St.
Austin, TX 78701
Contact: Kathryn Geiger, *Director of Medical Services*, Travis County Sheriff's Dept.
kathryn.geiger@traviscountytx.gov
512-854-4664
www.tcsheriff.org

In a unique partnership that was the brainchild of Sheriff Gregg Hamilton, the Travis County Sheriff's Dept. joined forces with the Texas Laser & Aesthetics Training Academy to create a traveling tattoo removal program within the Travis County Jail's medical facility in Austin, Texas. It was launched in September 2015.

Currently, the laser academy's co-owner and one of its head instructors offer their time for free to travel to the prison every other week. They take a portable tattoo removal device and spend six hours removing tattoos from about 25 patients.

The program is publicized in the prison's programs area, where inmates go for GED and work readiness classes, and anyone can participate. No one is turned away, but there is a waiting list.

The week before the procedures are performed, the Travis County Jail requires that participants undergo a physical examination by the prison's medical provider to make sure that their body is capable of absorbing the dye. And if they're on any medicines that make them photo sensitive, they'll need to stop those seven days before the procedure.

The prison's medical staff also requires those who receive treatment to come back the following day to meet with a wound care specialist, who ensures that the tattoo removal site is healing properly. Patients are also reminded to avoid the sun and keep the area moist with antibiotic cream.

Free follow-up sessions can be scheduled post release. These take place at the laser academy, where former inmates have their tattoos removed by its students.

Covering 'em up

It may take a while to put a tattoo removal program together, but in the meantime you can get a head start—or even establish a parallel program—by creating classes in using makeup to cover up tattoos. It's cheap, it's effective, and it works.

The idea came from a Baltimore nonprofit we contacted thinking they had a tattoo removal program. They don't. Instead they use a different method of dealing with visible tattoos, one they discovered in a totally serendipitous way.

It all began a couple of years ago, when the Ex-Offender Mentoring Academy and Training Center at Living Classrooms Foundation decided to work on family reunification with fathers who were newly released from prison and used face painting as a way to bring the dads and their kids together.

"We were talking with the face painter, and she said makeup is good for everything. It even covers up tattoos," said Howard Wicker, the center's director. "It covers up everything no matter what the skin color."

She said that they could wear makeup over their tattoos when they went to interviews. Wicker asked her if she would be willing to come in and teach his guys, almost entirely African-American, how to do it. She agreed.

And now the program has two makeup artists who come in on Saturdays on a regular basis to teach the clients how to cover up visible tattoos with makeup. "Our staff is on the lookout for someone with tattoos that jump out at you. Guys are putting tattoos right in the middle of their forehead," Wicker said. "We ask them to attend a session, and most of them do."

Wicker said organizations can find a makeup artist to do the same thing for their clients by getting in touch with a local community theater. They exist in every city and even some small towns. Find out the name and contact of their makeup artist—every community theater has one. Contact them to see if they'd be interested in teaching formerly gang-involved, and previously incarcerated, men and women with tattoos how to cover them up.

The makeup artists' skills are really being used, according to Wicker, and they are very much appreciated, because what they do can make a big difference in the lives of previously incarcerated people who are looking for work.

His organization buys the makeup but asks the guys they give it to to use it sparingly—only for interviews.

If you don't have the resources or time to set up such a program, you can refer individuals to a professional makeup artist—maybe you can find someone to donate their time—for a private session. Clients can also learn how to cover up tattoos with makeup by searching online, where articles on the subject, YouTube how-to videos and makeup recommendations can be found.

You can check out a couple of examples of instructional videos. One is done by a trainer at Napoleon Perdis Makeup Academy and can be found at: www.youtube.com/watch?v=IsuhuLg-p2I.

Another was created by an Australian who goes by the name of Nibbles and can be found at: www.youtube.com/watch?v=0K_L4EaFLrc. And they're both pretty impressive.

Other services to offer

Creating a free or low-cost tattoo removal program offers organizations an opportunity to reach their target audience with a variety of other services, if they so desire. It may be enough to just do tattoo removal procedures, but depending on the needs of the community, they might want to provide more.

Some of the organizations that already do this turn the tattoo removal sessions into an event. They recruit other providers who may be able to help those who come to get their tattoos removed with needs in other areas of their lives.

What can be done depends on the community, the resources and the desire of the sponsor organization. Possibilities include recruiting nonprofits or volunteers who can help with resume writing and job search assistance, other medical needs, dental care, education (GED information, for example), mentorship programs or any other services that might be appropriate.

Please feel free to visit our website at www.jailstojobs.org for advice, tips and resources, including downloadable handouts that support those with barriers to employment as they search for a job.

Your feedback is critical

We want to make the work we do as relevant and useful as possible to those developing and running tattoo removal programs. The only way we can do that is with your feedback. We'd like to know which of the things we wrote about in this book are most helpful and if there is anything we didn't include that you feel you need to know. Please send an email with your comments to info@jailstojobs.org.

If you or anyone you know would like to support our work, please visit www.jailstojobs.org and make a donation. We would be grateful if you did.

Jails to Jobs national directory of free and low-cost tattoo removal programs

This national directory of more than 200 free and low-cost tattoo removal programs in 37 states was developed primarily from hundreds of hours of Internet research and submitted programs. Some of them charge. Others are free but may have requirements. It is a work in progress and is by no means a complete list. Obviously, programs can come and go. Always contact any program you're interested in to confirm its criteria and requirements, including possible age restrictions, fees if any, and what may be required of client to obtain services. Always try and make contact first by telephone or email, as most programs work by appointment only.

Our most current directory is available at our website. If you would like your program added or know of a program that should be included, please submit the name and contact information at www.jailstojobs.org.

Alabama

There are no programs that we know of currently in this state, but if anyone is interested in starting one, please recommend this guide or tell them to contact us at info@jailstojobs.org.

Alaska

There are no programs that we know of currently in this state, but if anyone is interested in starting one, please recommend this guide or tell them to contact us at info@jailstojobs.org.

Arizona

MAB Tatts
Phoenix, AZ
480-695-2163 or 602-574-2177
www.mabtatts.com
Fee: Sliding Scale
Age Restrictions: Unknown
Call for eligibility and application. Service is designed to help people from all walks of life.

X-TATTOO
2039 S. Mill Ave.
Tempe, AZ 85281
Contact: Elizabeth McCowin
480-306-4198
www.xtattooremoval.com
Fee: Unknown
Age Restrictions: Unknown

Arizona (cont'd)

Dr. Tattoff
740 S. Mill Ave., Suite 130
Tempe, AZ 85281
Contact: Carol Mendelsohn, *Dir. of Marketing*
carol.mendelsohn@drtattoff.com
480-525-9238
www.drtattoff.com
Fee: 25% off a Tattoo Removal Package –
Mention Jails to Jobs
Age Restrictions: None

Arizona Laser Skin Solutions
The Tattoo Removal Clinic
512 E. Southern Ave, Suite D
Tempe, AZ 85282
Contact: Kevin Crawford, RN, FNP, *Owner*
480-921-0767
www.arizonalaser.com
Fee: None
Age Restrictions: Unknown

Arkansas

There are no programs that we know of currently in this state, but if anyone is interested in starting one, please recommend this guide or tell them to contact us at info@jailstojobs.org.

California

Clean Arms For Community
1175 East Lincoln Ave.
Anaheim, CA 92805
Contact: Taizo Shibayama
877-828-3233
www.cleanarms.org
Fee: None
Age Restrictions: Juveniles

Tattoo Vanish
1111 Dunbar Rd., #B-100
Arnold, CA 95223
Contact: Colleen Brohy
209-795-6795
Fee: Free tattoo removal for gang dropouts
and victims of human trafficking.
Age Restrictions: None

Agape Light Tattoo Removal Program
1331 3rd St.
Bakersfield, CA 93304
Contact: Ray or Maxine Patrick
661-863-0681
Fee: None –Sliding Scale
Age Restrictions: Unknown

Take Away Tattoos, Probation Auxiliary
County of Kern (P.A.C.K.)
2005 Ridge Rd.
Bakersfield, CA 93305
Contact: Elaine Moore, *Supervisor*
elainemoore@co.kern.ca.us
661-868-4159
www.kernprobation.com/pack
Fee: Unknown
Age Restrictions: Unknown

Bakersfield Eye Institute
7508 Meany Ave.
Bakersfield, CA 93308
661-589-9400
Fee: Unknown
Age Restrictions: Unknown

Beautologie Laser Center
Milan Shah, M.D.
4850 Commerce Dr.
Bakersfield, CA 93308
661-865-5009
www.beautologie.com
Fee: Unknown
Age Restrictions: Unknown

California (cont'd)

Stuart Kaplan, M.D.
435 North Roxbury Dr., Suite 210
Beverly Hills, CA 90210
310-858-7880
www.skindoc.net
Fee: Sliding Scale
Age Restrictions: None

Dr. Tattoff
8500 Wilshire Blvd., Suite 105
Beverly Hills, CA 90211
Contact: Carol Mendelsohn, *Dir. of Marketing*
carol.mendelsohn@drtattoff.com
310-659-5101
www.drtattoff.com
Fee: 25% off a Tattoo Removal Package–
Mention Jails to Jobs
Age Restrictions: None

One Day At a Time
331 Pine St.
Brentwood, CA 94513
Contact: Johnny Rodriquez
925-240-1359
www.odatec.org
Fee: None, must participate in their program
Age Restrictions: Juveniles–High School

Metamorphosis Medical Center
8081 Stanton Ave., Suite 300
Buena Park, CA 90620
714-484-8000
www.metamedcenter.com
Fee: Unknown
Age Restrictions: Unknown

Providence Saint Joseph Medical Center Community Outreach Center
501 South Buena Vista St.
Burbank, CA 91505
818-847-3860
http://california.providence.org/our-services/
tattoo-removal
Fee: Unknown
Age Restrictions: Unknown

Laser Away Tattoo Removal Clinic
6965 El Camino Real, Suite 104
Carlsbad, CA 92009
760-929-9944
www.laseraway.net
Fee: Unknown
Age Restrictions: Unknown

Donald Richey, M.D.
North Valley Dermatology Center
251 Cohasset Rd., Suite 240
Chico, CA 95926
530-342-3686
www.nvdermatology.com
Fee: Unknown
Age Restrictions: Unknown

Arrowhead Regional Medical Center, Gang Response and intervention Program (GRIP)
400 North Pepper Ave.
Colton, CA 92324
Contact: Winona Eichner
909-580-1669
www.arrowheadmedcenter.org
Fee: Unknown
Age Restrictions: Unknown

Tat2BeGone
420 N. McKinley St.
Corona, CA 92879
951-273-9911
www.tat2begone.com
Fee: Unknown
Age Restrictions: Unknown

California (cont'd)

Laser & Dermatology Institute of California
246 West College St., 3rd Floor
Covina, CA 91723
800-606-6000
www.laserhq.com
Fee: Free consultation. Sliding Scale
Age Restrictions: None

Kaiser Permanente
Right Turn Program
9449 East Imperial Highway
Downey, CA 90242
Contact: Onnie Lange
562-461-6081
Fee: Unknown
Age Restrictions: Unknown

EC Medical Group
127 East Lexington Ave., Suite F
El Cajon, CA 92020
Contact: Nina
619-447-1502
Fee: Sliding Scale
Age Restrictions: 18 years and under

El Monte Police Department
Tattoo Removal Service
11333 East Valley Blvd.
El Monte, CA 91731
Contact: Julie Soldana
626-580-2186
http://crg.lacounty.gov/dmh/ViewDetail.
aspx?ID=1000809001
Fee: None
Age Restrictions: 18 years and older

Washington Hospital
Tattoo Removal Program
2000 Mowry Ave.
Fremont, CA 94538
Contact: Lucy Hernandez
510-494-7009
www.whhs.com/community/tattoo-removal-
program/
Fee: None 24 years or younger, one-time fee 25
years and older, sliding scale.
Age Restrictions: Unknown

San Joaquin County Probation
Tattoo Removal Program
535 West Matthews Rd.
French Camp, CA 95231
Contact: Cynthia Bulmer
209-468-5539
www.sjgov.org/probation/JuvenileProb.
aspx?id=6260
Fee: None
Age Restrictions: Unknown

Beautologie Laser Center
1903 E. Fir Ave.
Fresno, CA 93720
559-476-4460
www.beautologie.com
Fee: None
Age Restrictions: Unknown

Hope Now for Youth, Inc.
2305 Stanislaus St.
Fresno, CA 93721
Contact: Dave Maravilla
559-237-7215
www.hopenowforyouth.org
Fee: None
Age Restrictions: 16–24 years old

California (cont'd)

City of Fresno
Mayor's Gang Prevention Initiative
2323 Mariposa St., Room 212
Fresno, CA 93721
Contact: Maggie Navarro, *Communications Coordinator*
Maggie.navarro@fresno.gov
559-621-2353
www.fresno.gov/Government/
DepartmentDirectory/Police/AboutFresnoPD/
PoliceServicesandSpecialUnits/
MayorsGangPreventionInitiative.htm
Fee: Unknown
Age Restrictions: Unknown

Pentecostal Church of God
323 East 11th St.
Hanford, CA 93230
559-582-1210
www.hanfordpc.com
Fee: Unknown
Age Restrictions: Unknown

Clean Slate, Hawaiian Gardens Community
22150 Wardhom Ave.
Hawaiian Gardens, CA 90716
Contact: Sylvia Gooden
562-945-9111
www.cleanslatela.org
Fee: Unknown
Age Restrictions: Unknown

Hayward New Start
Eden Youth Center
680 West Tennyson Road
Hayward, CA 94544
Contact: Cindy Gallegos
510-785-6690
www.acphd.org/project-new-start/contact-info.aspx
Fee: None. 50 hours of community service
Age Restrictions: 13–25 years old

UC Irvine Medical Center
Tattoo Removal Program
1002 Health Sciences Rd.
Irvine, CA 92617
Contact: Ruth Bundy
949-824-7997
www.bli.uci.edu
Fee: Varies
Age Restrictions: None

Church of Glad Tidings
1179 Eager Rd.
Live Oak, CA 95953
530-671-3160
www.churchofgladtidings.com
Fee: Unknown
Age Restrictions: Unknown

Loma Linda University Medical Center
Tattoo Removal Clinic
11234 Anderson St.
Loma Linda, CA 92354
909-558-7045
Fee: Unknown
Age Restrictions: Unknown

City of Long Beach Gang Intervention/
Prevention Tattoo Removal
1550 Martin Luther King Jr. Ave.
Long Beach, CA 90813
562-570-7260
Fee: Unknown
Age Restrictions: 14–24 years old

Erase the Past Tattoo Removal
Long Beach Police Department
333 West Broadway
Long Beach, CA 90802
Contact: Sandee Conn
562-818-9950
www.erasethepast.org
www.memorialcare.org/classes/class-details.cfm?id=402
Fee: Unknown
Age Restrictions: Unknown

California (cont'd)

A New Way of Life
836 E. 91st St.
Los Angeles, CA 90002
323-563-3575
www.anewwayoflife.org
Fee: Unknown
Age Restrictions: Unknown

Homeboy Industries
130 West Bruno St.
Los Angeles, CA 90012
Contact: Esmeralda Mendez,
Tattoo Removal Manager
emendez@homeboyindustries.org
323-526-1254, ext. 344
www.homeboyindustries.org
Fee: None
Age Restrictions: Unknown

Los Angeles County Sheriff's Pre-release Tattoo
Removal Program–Medical Services Bureau
450 Bauchet St., Room E873
Los Angeles, CA 90012
Contact: Alicia McKenzie
213-893-5445
http://shq.lasdnews.net/pages/PageDetail.
aspx?id=1395
Fee: Unknown
Age Restrictions: Unknown

Aztecs Rising
Public Health Foundation Enterprise, Inc.
1316 S. Union Ave.
Los Angeles, CA 90015
213-738-0178
www.aztecsrising.org
Fee: Unknown
Age Restrictions: Unknown

2nd Call
P.O. Box 191476
Los Angeles, CA 90019
310-916-1902
Contact: Skipp Townsend
www.2ndcall.org
Fee: Unknown
Age Restrictions: Unknown

City of Los Angeles, Mayor's Office
Gang Reduction & Youth Development
200 N. Spring, Room 303
Los Angeles, CA 90019
Contact: Nancy Avila, *Administrative Asst.*
213-473-7796
www.grydfoundation.org
Fee: Unknown
Age Restrictions: Unknown

Clean Slate Tattoo Removal, Inc.
5615 West Pico Blvd.
Los Angeles, CA 90019
Contact: Marianne Diaz
562-945-9111
www.cleanslatela.org
Fee: Negotiable, sliding scale
Age Restrictions: Unknown

B.U.I.L.D.
1409 W. Vernon Ave.
Los Angeles, CA 90026
Contact: Aquil Basheer, *Executive Director*
323-275-1904
www.maximumforceenterprises.org
Fee: Unknown
Age Restrictions: Unknown

Hollywood Sunset Free Clinic
3324 West Sunset Blvd.
Los Angeles, CA 90026
323-660-2400 or 323-660-7975, removal line
www.hsfreeclinic.org
Fee: Unknown
Age Restrictions: Unknown

California (cont'd)

Ya Estuvo Tattoo Removal Program
1916 East First St.
Los Angeles, CA 90033
323-526-0708
Fee: Unknown
Age Restrictions: Unknown

Clean Slate Tattoo Removal Program
White Memorial Medical Center
1720 Cesar Chavez Ave., Suite 1514
Los Angeles, CA 90033
323-268-5000
www.whitememorial.com
Fee: Negotiable, $50 per square inch
Age Restrictions: Unknown

Sunrise Outreach Tattoo Removal Clinic
Sunrise Community Outreach Center
2105 Beverly Blvd.
Los Angeles, CA 90057
Contact: Maria
213-483-2655
www.sunriseoutreach.org
Fee: $30–$100 per session
Age Restrictions: None

Homies Unidos
Epiphany Project
2105 Beverly Blvd., Suite 219
Los Angeles, CA 90057
Contact: Alejandro Alvardo
aalvardo@homiesunidos.org
213-383-7484
www.homiesunidos.org
Fee: Unknown
Age Restrictions: None

Martin Luther King Jr., Drew Medical Center
Tattoo Removal Program
12021 Wilmington Ave.
Los Angeles, CA 90059
310-668-4205
www.ladhs.org/wps/portal/KingHomepage
Fee: $50 consultation, $50 per treatment
Age Restrictions: Unknown

Agape Light Tattoo Removal Program
Culver City Seventh-Day Adventist Church
11828 West Washington Blvd.
Los Angeles, CA 90066
Contact: Pastor Jan Kart
310-398-9205
http://culvercity.adventistfaith.org
Fee: Unknown
Age Restrictions: Unknown

Steven Popkow, M.D.
Skin Laser Center
12027 Venice Blvd., Suite B
Los Angeles, CA 90066
310-915-8060
www.tattooremoval.org
Fee: Free consultation, sliding scale
Age Restrictions: Unknown

Juvenile Hall Auxiliary of Contra Costa County
202 Glacier Dr.
Martinez, CA 94553
Contact: Janet Young, *Executive Director*
janet@reachingouryouth.org
925-957-2718
www.reachingouryouth.org
Fee: Unknown
Age Restrictions: Unknown

California (cont'd)

Providence Holy Cross Medical Center
Tattoo Removal Clinic
15031 Rinaldi St.
Mission Hills, CA 91345
818-898-4416
https://california.providence.org/HolyCross/
pages/tattoo.aspx
Fee: None, donations accepted
Age Restrictions: Unknown

Skin Renew Laser Medical Center
1213 Coffee Rd., Suite Q
Modesto, CA 95355
209-526-2200
www.skinrenewmedical.com
Fee: Unknown
Age Restrictions: Unknown

Dr. Tattoff
9197 Central Ave., Suite H
Montclair, CA 91763
Contact: Carol Mendelsohn, *Dir. of Marketing*
carol.mendelsohn@drtattoff.com
909-267-7200
www.drtattoff.com
Fee: 25% off a Tattoo Removal Package–
Mention Jails to Jobs
Age Restrictions: None

Taboo Tattoo Removal Program at Wolfe
Center, Aldea Behavioral Health Services
2310 First St.
Napa, CA 94559
Contact: Anna Hernandez, *Program Director*
707-255-1855
www.aldeainc.org
Fee: Unknown
Age Restrictions: Unknown

Second Chance, Inc.
New Beginnings (Tattoo Removal)
P.O. Box 643
Newark, CA 94560
www.secondchanceinc.com
510-886-8696
Fee: Unknown
Age Restrictions: Unknown
Apply by telephone

Communities in Schools (CIS) of the
San Fernando Valley & Greater Los Angeles
8743 Burnet Ave.
North Hills, CA 91343
Contact: Nicole Rivera
818-891-9399
www.cisgla.org
Fee: None
Age Restrictions: Unknown

Project New Start, Alameda County
Public Health Department
1000 Broadway, 5th Floor
Oakland, CA 94607
Contact: Adriana Alvarado
510-383-5217
www.acphd.org/project-new-start.aspx
Fee: None
Age Restrictions: 13–25 years

Butte County Probation Department
Tattoo Removal Program
2279 Del Oro Ave.
Oroville, CA 95965
Contact: Marina Aldridge
530-538-7661
www.buttecounty.net/probation
Fee: Unknown
Age Restrictions: Unknown

California (cont'd)

Las Islas Familia Clinic
Santa Paula Tattoo Removal Program
2400 S. C St.
Oxnard, CA 93035
Contact: Martin Hernandez, *Clinic Coordinator*
Martin.Hernandez@ventura.org
805-654-2276
www.vchca.org
Fee: 40 hours of community service or cash
donation
Age Restrictions: None

Gang Intervention Team (G.R.I.T.)
101 E. Redlands Blvd., Suite 203
Redlands, CA 92374
Contact: Joseph Rodriguez
grityouthservices@hotmail.com
909-793-7746
www.grityouthservices.com
Fee: Unknown
Age Restrictions: Unknown

San Mateo County Tattoo Removal Program
Redwood City PAL Community Center
3399 Bay Rd.
Redwood City, CA 94063
Contact: Manual Velarde
mvelarde@redwoodcity.org
650-780-7100 ext. 7195
www.redwoodcitypal.com/programs/tattoo
Fee: None
Age Restrictions: Unknown

Riverside County
Department of Community Action
2038 Iowa Ave., Suite B-102
Riverside, CA 92507
951-955-4900
www.capriverside.org
Fee: Unknown
Age Restrictions: 19 years and under

Emil A. Tanghetti, M.D.
Laser Surgery Center
5601 "J" St.
Sacramento, CA 95819
916-454-5922
www.dermatologyandlasersurgery.com
Fee: Unknown–Discounted rates if referred by
Youth Authority from surrounding counties.
Age Restrictions: Unknown

Inkoff.me
5534 Elvas Ave.
Sacramento, CA 95819
Contact: Chris Bendinelli
chris@inkoff.me
916-600-4428
www.inkoff.me
Fee: Unknown
Age Restrictions: None

2nd Chance Family & Youth Services
745 North Sanborn Rd.
Salinas, CA 93906
Contact: Reuben Urvua
831-758-2501
www.scyp.org
Fee: $50 orientation fee or 20 hours of community
service–Plus $25 per session and 20 hours
community service.
Age Restrictions: 25 years and under

Family Health Centers of San Diego
823 Gateway Center Way
San Diego, CA 92102
619-515-2366
www.fhcsd.org
Fee: Unknown
Age Restrictions: Unknown

Laser Away Tattoo Removal (Downtown)
3739 Sixth Ave.
San Diego, CA 92103
619-295-2929
Fee: Unknown
Age Restrictions: Unknown

California (cont'd)

United African American Ministerial Action Council
404 Euclid Ave., Suite 378
San Diego, CA 92114
619-264-1213
www.uaamac.org
Fee: Unknown
Age Restrictions: Unknown

Laser Clinic Tattoo Removal (Pacific Beach)
3737 Moraga Ave., Suite B-214
San Diego, CA 92117
858-272-2021
Fee: Unknown
Age Restrictions: Unknown

Rise Up Industries
San Diego, CA
Contact: Joe Gilbreath
j.gilbreath@riseupindustries.org
619-354-8460
www.riseupindustries.org
Fee: $60 per session
Age Restrictions: Minors require parental approval

Laser Away Tattoo Removal (UTC)
8935 Towne Center Dr., Suite 107A
San Diego, CA 92122
858-452-2929
Fee: Unknown
Age Restrictions: Unknown

San Francisco General Hospital Children's Health Center
1001 Potrero Ave., 6th Floor
San Francisco, CA 94110
415-206-8376
www.sfdph.org
Fee: None, donations accepted
Age Restrictions: 25 years and under

TattooBeGoneSF
Serenity Med Spa
77 Maiden Lane, 2nd Floor
San Francisco, CA 94108
415-766-0625
www.serenitymedspa.com/laser-tattoo-removal-san-francisco
Fee: Unknown
Age Restrictions: Unknown

Second Chance Tattoo Removal
Central American Resource Center (CARECEN)
3101 Mission St.
San Francisco, CA 94110
Contact: Vanessa
415-642-4400
www.carecensf.org
Fee: None
Age Restrictions: 12–24 years

Clean Slate Tattoo Removal Program
1694 Adrian Way
San Jose, CA 95122
Contact: Jose Avila or Raul Perez
408-794-1660
www.sanjoseca.gov
Fee: Unknown
Age Restrictions: 14–25 years

New Skin Adult Tattoo Removal
1060 Willow St.
San Jose, CA 95125
Contact: Adam King, *Executive Director*
adam.king@newskinadulttattooremoval.org
408-899-9695
www.newskintr.org
Fee: $50 per session
Age Restrictions: None

California (cont'd)

Liberty Tattoo Removal Program
Sierra Vista Regional Medical Center
1010 Murray Ave.
San Luis Obispo, CA 93405
Contact: Janet Allenspach
805-544-2484 or 805-544-5033
www.sierravistaregional.com
Fee: 16 hours of community service per session
Age Restrictions: None

Removing Barriers
San Pablo Economic Development Corporation
13830 San Pablo Ave., Suite D
San Pablo, CA 94806
Contact: Leslay Choy, *Executive Director*
leslayc@sanpabloedc.org
510-215-3189
www.sanpabloedc.org
Fee: San Pablo residents $50 per session and
non-residents $80 per session.
Age Restrictions: None

Orange County Probation Dept., Tattoo
Removal Program at St. Joseph's Hospital
909 N. Main St.
Santa Ana, CA 92701
714-569-3796
www.ocgov.com/gov/probation/employment/
volunteer/pcaa
Fee: Unknown
Age Restrictions: Unknown

Dr. Tattoff
1441 West MacArthur Blvd., Suite A
Santa Ana, CA 92704
Contact: Carol Mendelsohn, *Dir. of Marketing*
carol.mendelsohn@drtattoff.com
949-581-5334
www.drtattoff.com
Fee: 25% off a Tattoo Removal Package–
Mention Jails to Jobs
Age Restrictions: None

Laser Medical Center
3816 Bristol St., Suite M
Santa Ana, CA 92704
Contact: Russ Calendar
714-662-7456
www.lasermed4skin.com
Fee: Sliding Scale
Age Restrictions: Unknown

Liberty Program
American Indian Health & Services
4141 State St., Suite B-2
Santa Barbara, CA 93110
805-681-7356 ext. 223
www.aihscorp.org/programs/liberty-program
Fee: None
Age Restrictions: Unknown

City of Santa Clarita
23920 Valencia Blvd., Suite 300
Santa Clarita, CA 91355
Contact: Cynthia llerenes
661-286-4006 ext. 5057
http://user.govoutreach.com/santaclarita/faq.
php?cid=6673
Fee: Unknown
Age Restrictions: Unknown

Catholic Charities of the Diocese of Monterey
610 Frederick St.
Santa Cruz, 95062
charities.trp@catholiccharitiescentralcoast.org
831-431-6939
www.catholiccharitiescentralcoast.org
Fee: $20 per session with a sliding scale.
Age Restrictions: None

California (cont'd)

Santa Paula Tattoo Removal Project
1334 E. Main St.
Santa Paula, CA 93060
Contact: Martin Hernandez, *Clinic Coordinator*
Martin.Hernandez@ventura.org
805-933-1242
www.vchca.org
Fee: 40 hours community service or cash donation
Age Restrictions: None

Santa Rosa Violence Prevention Partnership Tattoo Removal Program, Rec. & Parks Dept.
415 Steele Lane
Santa Rosa, CA 95404
Contact: Khaalid Muttaqi, *Program Manager*
707-543-3457
www.santarosarec.com
Fee: Unknown
Age Restrictions: Unknown

Dr. Tattoff
13833 Ventura Blvd., Suite 103
Sherman Oaks, CA 91423
Contact: Carol Mendelsohn, *Dir. of Marketing*
carol.mendelsohn@drtattoff.com
818-907-9200
www.drtattoff.com
Fee: 25% off a Tattoo Removal Package–
Mention Jails to Jobs
Age Restrictions: None

San Mateo County Probation Department
1024 Mission Rd.
South San Francisco, CA 94080
Contact: John Domeniconi
650-312-8816
Fee: Unknown
Age Restrictions: Unknown

Inkoff.me
1151 West Robinhood Dr., Suite B14
Stockton, CA 95207
Contact: Chris Bendinelli
chris@inkoff.me
916-600-4428
www.inkoff.me
Fee: Unknown
Age Restrictions: None

Friends Outside
7272 Murray Dr.
Stockton, CA 95210
Contact: John Medina, *Reentry and Event Coordinator*
jmedina@friendsoutside.org
209-955-0701
www.friendsoutside.org
Fee: None
Age Restrictions: Unknown

Allure Image Enhancement, Inc.
1113 Alta Ave., Suite 210
Upland, CA 91786
909-982-1074
www.allureimage.com
Fee: Unknown
Age Restrictions: Unknown

Only Skin Deep
622 Tuolomne St.
Vallejo, CA 94590
707-642-1961
Fee: Unknown
Age Restrictions: Unknown

California (cont'd)

Creekside Laser Center
2820 West Main St.
Visalia, CA 93291
559-625-2737
www.creeksidedayspa.com
Fee: Unknown
Age Restrictions: Unknown

Agape Light Tattoo Removal
Thomas F. Mitts, M.D., Inc.
205 South West St., Suite A
Visalia, CA 93291
559-625-4234
www.drmitts.com
Fee: Unknown
Age Restrictions: Unknown

Pacific Union Church Support Services
P.O. Box 5005
Westlake Village, CA 91359
805-413-7372
www.churchsupportservices.org
Fee: Unknown
Age Restrictions: Unknown

Clean Slate
WRHAP Youth Center
12401 East Slauson Ave.
Whittier, CA 90606
Contact: Marianne Diaz
323-937-1344 ext. 3211
www.cleanslatela.org
Fee: Unknown
Age Restrictions: Unknown

Colorado

Aurora's Gang Reduction Impact Program
(A-GRIP)
7375 S. Potomac St.
Aurora, CO 80112
Contact: Shawn Barrett
720-874-3381
www.jac18.org
Fee: Unknown
Age Restrictions: Unknown

Tattoo Undo
8719 E. Dry Creek Rd., Suite B
Centennial, CO 80112
303-990-0120
www.tattooundo.net
Fee: Unknown
Age Restrictions: Unknown

Gang Rescue and Support Project
GRASP is a program of Metro Denver Partners
701 Logan St., Suite 109
Denver, CO 80209
303-777-3117
www.graspyouth.org
Fee: Unknown
Age Restrictions: Unknown

What Were You Inking?
2544 15th St.
Denver, CO 80211
Contact: Jill France, *Owner*
303-455-5900
www.whatwereyouinking.com
Fee: Free to ex-offenders of the Colorado
Department of Corrections.
Age Restrictions: Unknown

Colorado (cont'd)

Longmont Children, Youth & Families
Gang Response and Intervention Program
(GRIP)
1050 Lashley St..
Longmont, CO 80504
Contact: Louie Lopez, *Community Coordinator*
louie.lopez@longmontcolorado.gov
303-774-3756
www.longmontcolorado.gov/departments/
departments-a-d/children-youth-and-families
Fee: $50
Age Restrictions: 11–19 years

Connecticut

Connecticut Skin Institute
999 Summer St., #305
Stamford, CT 06905
info@ctskindoc.com
203-428-4440
www.ctskindoc.com
Fee: Unknown
Age Restrictions: Unknown

Delaware

There are no programs that we know of currently
in this state, but if anyone is interested in starting
one, please recommend this guide or tell them to
contact us at info@jailstojobs.org.

Florida

Jacksonville Re-Entry Center (JREC)
1024 Superior St.
Jacksonville, FL 32254
904-301-2400
www.coj.net/departments/sheriffs-office/
department-of-corrections/prisons-division/
jacksonville-reentry-center-(jrec).aspx
Fee: Unknown
Age Restrictions: Unknown

Miami Tattoo Company
1218 Washington Ave.
Miami, FL 33139
miamitattoocosobe@gmail.com
305-531-0204
www.miamitattooco.com
Fee: Free to victims of human trafficking.
Age Restrictions: Unknown

Fresh Start Tattoo Removal Program, Inc.
"Beat the Ink"
9065 SW 87th Ave., Suite 109
Miami, FL 33176
305-271-7800
www.beattheink.com
Fee: Unknown
Age Restrictions: Unknown

Skin Deep Naples
5490 Bryson Dr., #202
Naples, FL 34109
239-249-8309
www.skindeepnaples.com
Fee: Free to former gang members.
Age Restrictions: Unknown

Georgia

Dr. Tattoff
3637 Peachtree Rd., Suite D-1
Atlanta, GA 30319
Contact: Carol Mendelsohn, *Dir. of Marketing*
carol.mendelsohn@drtattoff.com
404-490-4300
www.drtattoff.com
Fee: 25% off a Tattoo Removal Package–
Mention Jails to Jobs
Age Restrictions: Unknown

Georgia Boyz Ink Works
157 Central Dr., East
Dublin, GA 31027
Contact: Mark Martin
478-272-6944
Fee: Unknown
Age Restrictions: Unknown

Hawaii

Fresh Start Tattoo Removal Program, Inc.
Way Gone Tattoo Removal
320 Ward Ave., #210
Honolulu, HI 96814
808-721-6518
www.waygonelasertattooremoval.com
Fee: Unknown
Age Restrictions: Unknown

Idaho

Second Chance Grace Tattoo Removal
P.O. Box 1058
Meridian, ID 83680
Contact: Jeri Vasquez, *Program Manager*
jeri@2ndchancegrace.org
208-703-6930
www.2ndchancegrace.org
Fee: Under 18 years, no charge, Over 18 years $45
per session.
Age Restrictions: Unknown

Illinois

Cook County Jail
Pre-Trial Tattoo Removal Program
2700 California Ave.
Chicago, IL 60608
Contact: Cara Smith, *Executive Director,*
Cook County Jail
cara.smith@cookcounty.gov
773-674-7100
www.cookcountysheriff.org
Fee: None
Age Restrictions: None

Tattoo Removal Centers of America
2825 North Halsted St.
Chicago, IL 60657
855-863-6465
Fee: Unknown
Age Restrictions: Unknown

Corazon Community Services
2138 S 61st Ct.
Cicero, IL 60804
708-656-1400
www.corazoncs.org
Fee: Unknown
Age Restrictions: Unknown

Gang Outreach
P.O. Box 7857
Gurnee, IL 60031
847-727-9417
www.oocities.org/~gangoutreach/index.html
Fee: Unknown
Age Restrictions: Unknown

Ink 180 Mobile Tattoo Removal Program
27 Stonehill Rd., Unit D
Oswego, IL 60543
Contact: Chris Baker, *Chief Ink Officer*
Chris Baker: chris@ink180.com
630-554-1404
www.ink180.com
Fee: None, for former gang members and victims
of human trafficking.
Age Restrictions: Unknown

Indiana

Bugaboo Tattoo
7014 Kennedy Ave.
Hammond, IN 46323
Contact: Lenise Towarnicki
219-844-4343
www.bugabootattoo.com
Fee: None, for juveniles in the Lake County
system.
Age Restrictions: Unknown

Indiana (cont'd)

Indy Tattoo Removal, LLC
2010 West 86th St., Suite #100
Indianapolis, IN 46260
317-800-6600
www.indytattooremoval.com
Fee: Unknown
Age Restrictions: Unknown

Iowa

There are no programs that we know of currently in this state, but if anyone is interested in starting one, please recommend this guide or tell them to contact us at info@jailstojobs.org.

Kansas

AesthetiCare MedSpa
11100 Ash St.
Leawood, KS 66211
Contact: Matt Taranto
913-535-8916
www.greatskinkc.com
Fee: Up to 75% discount
Age Restrictions: Unknown

Wichita Crime Commission
Gang Tattoo Removal Program
300 North Main St., Suite 202
Wichita, KS 67202
Contact: John Biagini
316-267-1235
www.wichitacrimecommission.org/
gangfreewichita/default.aspx
Fee: Unknown
Age Restrictions: Unknown

Kentucky

There are no programs that we know of currently in this state, but if anyone is interested in starting one, please recommend this guide or tell them to contact us at info@jailstojobs.org.

Louisiana

There are no programs that we know of currently in this state, but if anyone is interested in starting one, please recommend this guide or tell them to contact us at info@jailstojobs.org.

Maine

Cosmetic Enhancement Center
Maria Atkins, D.O.
1375 Congress St.
Portland, ME 04102
207-761-0177
www.cecofne.com
Fee: No cost or very low cost.
Age Restrictions: Juveniles of Long Creek Youth Development.

Maryland

Identity, Inc.
Youth Opportunity Center
414 East Diamond Ave
Gaithersburg, MD 20877
301-591-1790
www.identity-youth.org
Fee: Unknown
Age Restrictions: Unknown

Massachusetts

Tataway Laser Tattoo Removal
123 South St., 4th Floor
Boston, MA 02111
Contact: Carmen Vanderheiden, *Owner*
857-284-4800
ww.tataway.com/outreach
Fee: None. Free tattoo removal on the hands, neck and face of those who were formerly incarcerated, former gang members, survivors of human trafficking or former sex workers.
Age Restrictions: None

Massachusetts (cont'd)

SkinCare Physicians
1244 Boylston St.
Chestnut Hill, MA 02467
Contact: Beth Hartigan
617-731-1600
www.skincarephysicians.net
Fee: Unknown
Age Restrictions: Unknown

Amirah, Inc.
P.O. Box 54
Wenham, MA 01984
781-462-1758
www.amirahboston.org
For victims of human trafficking.
Fee: Unknown
Age Restrictions: Unknown

Michigan

Detroit Hispanic Development Corporation
1211 Trumbull St.
Detroit, MI 48216
Contact: James Phillips
313-967-4880
www.dhdc1.org
Fee: $25 per session, sliding scale
Age Restrictions: Unknown

Dr. Eric Seiger, Freedom Ink Skin and Vein Center
32669 Warren Rd., #9
Garden City, MI 48135
734-762-0798
www.drericseiger.com
Fee: None
Age Restrictions: Unknown

Grand Rapids Tattoo Removal and Skin Clinic
1515 Michigan St. NE, Suite 125
Grand Rapids, MI 49525
Contact: Anthony Neilly, *C.L.T.*
616-403-1970
www.purebornskin.com
Fee: None
Age Restrictions: None

Minnesota

Fade Away Laser Tattoo Removal
10 East Superior St., #203
Duluth, MN 55802
218-720-3233
www.fadeawaylaser.com
Fee: Free to victims of sex trafficking.
Age Restrictions: None

Zel Skin and Laser Specialist
4100 West 50th St.
Edina, MN 55424
952-929-8888
www.zelskin.com
Fee: Sliding Scale
Age Restrictions: 18 years and older

Northeast Laser Tattoo Removal, LLC
924 Lowry Ave. NE
Minneapolis, MN 55418
Contact: Aleksandar Nedich or
Thomas H. Borrows, M.D., *Owners*
612-788-4100
www.nelasertattooremoval.com
Fee: Free to victims of human trafficking.
Age Restrictions: None

Highbridge Tattoo and Laser Removal
608 Smith Ave. S
Saint Paul, MN 55107
Contact: Aleksandar Nedich or
Thomas H. Borrows, M.D., *Owners*
651-330-1208
www.highbridgelaser.com
Fee: Free to victims of human trafficking.
Age Restrictions: None

Minnesota (cont'd)

Neighborhood House
GRIP
179 Robie St. East
Saint Paul, MN 55107
Contact: Enrique "Cha-Cho" Estrada
651-789-2500
www.neighb.org/programs/grip
Fee: Unknown
Age Restrictions: 12–25 years

Beloved Studios
1563 Como Ave.
Saint Paul, MN 55108
Contact: Vaness Lilke, *Certified Laser Technician,*
Brandon and Karis Heffron, *Owners*
651-255-3394
www.belovedstudios.com
Fee: Unknown
Age Restrictions: Unknown

Mississippi

There are no programs that we know of currently in this state, but if anyone is interested in starting one, please recommend this guide or tell them to contact us at info@jailstojobs.org.

Missouri

Under My Skin Tattoo Removal
500 North 3rd St., Suite C
Ozark, MO 65721
Contact: Amy Kern, *Owner*
akern@umstattooremoval.com
417-425-1788
www.umstattooremoval.com
Fee: Unknown
Age Restrictions: Unknown

On Second Thought Laser Tattoo Removal
2424 S. Campbell Ave., Suite 120
Springfield, MO 65907
Contact: Brian Kent, *Owner*
417-889-8408
www.springfieldtattooremoval.com
Fee: None for victims of human trafficking.
Age Restrictions: None

Plastic Surgery Consultants of Missouri
10004 Kennerly Rd., Suite 365B
St. Louis, MO 63128
314-842-5885
www.stl-psc.com
Fee: None
Age Restrictions: None

Vanishing Point Tattoo Removal
8601 Olive Blvd.
St. Louis, MO 63132
314-971-5297
www.vplaser.com
Fee: Discounted rates for the removal of tattoos for military enlistment, gang related tattoos, and free treatment of radiation tattoos.
Age Restrictions: None

Montana

Tallman Medical Spa
2294 Grant Rd.
Billings, MT 59102
406-294-9515
www.tallmanmedicalspa.com
Fee: Unknown
Age Restrictions: Unknown

Nebraska

Watchful Eye Foundation
1208 5th Ave.
South Sioux City, NE 68776
402-412-3393
Fee: None. Must participate in their program.
Age Restrictions: Juveniles

Nevada

Southern Nevada Community Gang Task Force
Clark County Juvenile Justice
601 N. Pecos
Las Vegas, NV 89155
Contact: Jerome Simon, *Gang Specialist*
simonje@co.clark.nv.us
702-455-2179
www.communitygangtaskforce.com
Fee: Unknown
Age Restrictions: Unknown

New Hampshire

There are no programs that we know of currently
in this state, but if anyone is interested in starting
one, please recommend this guide or tell them to
contact us at info@jailstojobs.org.

New Jersey

Fresh Start Tattoo Removal Program, Inc.
SOMA Skin & Laser Care
90 Millburn Ave., Suite 206
Millburn, NJ 07041
973-763-7546
www.somalaser.com
Fee: Unknown
Age Restrictions: Unknown

New Mexico

D-Ink
3939 San Pedro NE, Suite C7
Albuquerque, NM 87110
Contact: Dawn Maestas
505-220-6629
Fee: Unknown
Age Restrictions: Unknown

Clear Waves Medical Laser Group
1120 Juan Tabo Blvd. NE
Albuquerque, NM 87112
505-888-3733
www.clearwaves.com
Fee: 25% discount for ex-offenders.
Age Restrictions: Teens and adults only.

Tattoo Remorse
1650 Hospital Dr., Suite 800
Santa Fe, NM 87505
505-690-4919
www.tattooremorsesf.com
Fee: Unknown
Age Restrictions: Unknown

New York

Montefiore Medical Center
Cosmetic Dermatology Clinic
Karthik Krishnamurthy, D.O.
111 East 210th St.
Bronx, NY 10467
866-633-8255 x4801
www.montefiore.org/default.cfm?id=1
Fee: Sliding Scale
Age Restrictions: None

Fresh Start Tattoo Removal Program, Inc.
David J. Ores, M.D.
189 East 2nd St.
New York, NY 10009
917-723-4206
www.freshstarttattooremoval.org
Fee: Unknown
Age Restrictions: Unknown
See application at website.

New York (cont'd)

Tataway Laser Tattoo Removal
381 Park Ave. South, Suite 720
New York, NY 10016
Contact: Carmen Vanderheiden, *Owner*
857-284-4800
www.tataway.com/outreach
Fee: None. Free tattoo removal on the hands, neck
and face of those who were formerly incarcerated,
former gang members, survivors of human
trafficking or former sex workers.
Age Restrictions: None

Juva Skin and Laser Center
Bruce Katz, M.D.
60 East 56th St., Second Floor
New York, NY 10022
212-688-5882
www.juvaskin.com
Fee: None. Free with a $250 deposit which is
refunded at the completion of the procedures.
Age Restrictions: None

Fresh Start Tattoo Removal Program, Inc.
Clean Slate Laser
280 Mamaroneck Ave., Suite 208
White Plains, NY 10605
914-949-7943
www.cleanslatelaser.com
Fee: Unknown
Age Restrictions: Unknown

North Carolina

Vanish Ink
1315 East Blvd., Suite 190
Charlotte, NC 28204
Contact: Mark Biddy
704-334-0007
www.vanish-ink.com/index.htm
Fee: None, for gang related, discounted for minors.
Age Restrictions: None

Gang of ONE Program
200 E. Long Ave.
Gastonia, NC 28052
Contact: Patrick Daley, *Program Director*
704-864-7233
www.GO1gaston.org
Fee: None. Must participate in their program.
Age Restrictions: Juveniles

Carolina Laser & Cosmetic Center
45 Kimel Park, Suite 140
Winston Salem, NC 27103
336-659-2663
www.carolinalaser.com
Fee: None. Free, to all active military members
and veterans. Contact for details.
Age Restrictions: Unknown

North Dakota

Vanished Ink
118 North Broadway Dr., #521
Fargo, ND 58102
Contact: Keri Nybo or Renee Danielson, *Owners*
701-205-3871
www.vanishedink.com
Fee: Unknown
Age Restrictions: Unknown

Ohio

Advanced Cosmetic Surgery & Laser Center
Jon Mendelsohn, M.D.
Rockwood Commons Shopping Center
3805 Edwards Rd., #100
Cincinnati, OH 45209
513-351-3223
www.351face.com
Fee: None
Age Restrictions: Unknown

Ohio (cont'd)

Survivor's Ink
P.O. Box 9184
Columbus, OH 43209
Contact: Jennifer Kempton
survivors.ink2013@yahoo.com
www.survivorsink.org
Fee: Scholarships available for survivors of human trafficking and sexual exploitation.
Age Restrictions: Unknown

Oklahoma

There are no programs that we know of currently in this state, but if anyone is interested in starting one, please recommend this guide or tell them to contact us at info@jailstojobs.org.

Oregon

INK OUT
Valley Immediate Care
235 East Barnett Rd.
Medford, OR 97501
541-734-9030
www.pristinelaserservices.com/Ink-Out.html
Fee: Free or $25 tattoo removal to qualifying candidates referred by the Juvenile Justice Department.
Age Restrictions: Unknown

Outside In
1132 SW 13th Ave.
Portland, OR 97205
Contact: Tamara Bartlett
tamarab@outsidein.org
503-535-3902
www.outsidein.org/medical-services-tattoo-removal.htm
Fee: $25-$50 per session
Age Restrictions: Unknown

RediMedi Skin Clinics
1847 East Burnside St., Suite B
Portland, OR 97214
503-235-0782
www.redimediskinclinics.com
Fee: $25–$50 for every other session. Pay for one session and get the next session free.
Age Restrictions: Unknown

Oregon Youth Authority
Office of Inclusion and Intercultural Relations
Tattoo Removal Program
2450 Strong Rd. SE
Salem, OR 97302
503-986-0400
www.oregon.gov/oya
Fee: Unknown
Age Restrictions: Unknown

VIDA Aesthetic Medicine
1115 Liberty St. SE
Salem, OR 97302
Contact: Anita Wilbur
503-399-0021
www.vidaskincare.com
Fee: Unknown
Age Restrictions: Up to 19 years old.

Pennsylvania

Fresh Start Tattoo Removal Program, Inc.
Go Tattoo Removal
1011 Brookside Rd., #205
Allentown, PA 18106
484-648-0048
www.gotattooremoval.com
Fee: Unknown
Age Restrictions: Unknown

Pennsylvania (cont'd)

Tataway Laser Tattoo Removal
9 West 4th St.
Bethlehem, PA 18015
Contact: Carmen Vanderheiden, *Owner*
857-284-4800
www.tataway.com/outreach
Fee: None. Free tattoo removal on the hands, neck and face of those who were formerly incarcerated, former gang members, survivors of human trafficking or former sex workers.
Age Restrictions: None

Tataway Laser Tattoo Removal
16 South 3rd St.
Philadelphia, PA 19106
Contact: Carmen Vanderheiden, *Owner*
857-284-4800
www.tataway.com/outreach
Fee: None. Free tattoo removal on the hands, neck and face of those who were formerly incarcerated, former gang members, survivors of human trafficking or former sex workers.
Age Restrictions: None

East Side Laser Center
5770 Baum Blvd., Suite 200
Pittsburgh, PA 15206
412-363-7546
www.eastsidelasercenter.com
Fee: None
Age Restrictions: Unknown

Rhode Island

There are no programs that we know of currently in this state, but if anyone is interested in starting one, please recommend this guide or tell them to contact us at info@jailstojobs.org.

South Carolina

Richland County Gang Task Force
5623 Two Notch Rd.
Columbia, SC 29223
Contact: Leon Lott, *Sheriff*
803-518-1440
www.rcsd.net/comm/gangtask.htm
Fee: Unknown
Age Restrictions: Juveniles

South Dakota

T.R.U.S.T.
Tattoo Removal Unified Support Team
300 Kansas City St., Suite 400
Rapid City, SD 57701
Contact: Cody Raterman, *Program Director*
605-394-2191
www.pennco.org/index.asp?SEC=433072B4-E1B6-4648-BE17-0428AD8216C1&Type=B_Basic
Fee: None, must participate in their program
Age Restrictions: Juveniles

Tennessee

There are no programs that we know of currently in this state, but if anyone is interested in starting one, please recommend this guide or tell them to contact us at info@jailstojobs.org.

Texas

Fade Fast Laser Tattoo Removal
2928 Main St., Suite 100
Dallas, TX 75226
214-394-6824
www.fadefast.com
Fee: Unknown
Age Restrictions: Unknown

Texas (cont'd)

The Youth Removal Project
2928 Main St., Suite 100
Dallas, TX 75226
214-394-6824
www.youthremoval.org
Fee: No charge for gang related tattoos on head, neck, or face.
Age Restrictions: Under 18 years

Dr. Tattoff
11661 Preston Rd., Suite 128
Dallas, TX 75230
Contact: Carol Mendelsohn, *Dir. of Marketing*
carol.mendelsohn@drtattoff.com
469-547-6940
www.drtattoff.com
Fee: 25% off a Tattoo Removal Package– Mention Jails to Jobs
Age Restrictions: None

Dallas Tattoo Removal Clinic
8204 Elmbrook Dr., #117
Dallas, TX 75247
Contact: Mike or Glenda
214- 678-9550
www.dallastattooremovalclinic.biz
Fee: No fee if under 17 and tattoo is on hands or face. Otherwise $75 per session for 4″ x 4″ tattoos.
Age Restrictions: None

Travis County Correctional Complex
Pre-release Program
3614 Bill Price Rd.
Del Valle, TX 78617
512-854-9889
www.tcsheriff.org
Fee: None
Age Restrictions: Unknown

Project Bravo
Texas Youth Commission
9600 Dyer
El Paso, TX 79924
915-298-9600
www.projectbravo.org/language/english/
directory/texas-youth-commision
Fee: $25 per three sessions.
Age Restrictions: Unknown

D-Tag Tattoo Removal Program
Metrocrest Medical Foundation
One Medical Parkway, Suite 202
Farmers Branch, TX 75234
Contact: Cia Bond, *Executive Director*
cbond@mmftx.org
972-247-0286
www.mmftx.org/dtag.html
Fee: Unknown
Age Restrictions: Unknown

Dr. Tattoff
2600 West 7th St., Suite 104
Fort Worth, TX 76107
Contact: Carol Mendelsohn, *Dir. of Marketing*
carol.mendelsohn@drtattoff.com
682-730-8399
www.drtattoff.com
Fee: 25% off a Tattoo Removal Package– Mention Jails to Jobs
Age Restrictions: None

Dr. Tattoff
3401 Preston Rd., Suite D-6
Frisco, TX 75034
Contact: Carol Mendelsohn, *Dir. of Marketing*
carol.mendelsohn@drtattoff.com
469-296-4988
www.drtattoff.com
Fee: 25% off a Tattoo Removal Package– Mention Jails to Jobs
Age Restrictions: None

Texas (cont'd)

Giddings State School
Texas Juvenile Justice Department
2261 James Turman Rd.
P.O. Box 600
Giddings, TX 78942
979-542-4500
Fee: Unknown
Age Restrictions: Unknown

D-Tag Tattoo Removal Program
Harris County Medical Society
1515 Hermann Dr.
Houston, TX 77004
Contact: Emily Broussard
832-395-7297
www.hcms.org/about/Dtag
Fee: Unknown
Age Restrictions: 24 years and under

New Look Laser Tattoo Removal
19 Briar Hollow Lane, Suite 115
Houston, TX 77027
Contact@NewLookHouston.com
713-322-7304
www.newlookhouston.com
Fee: None, for gang-related tattoos on the face, hands, and neck.
Age Restrictions: Unknown

Houston Tattoo Removal Clinic
12841 Gulf Freeway
Houston, TX 77034
281-922-4262
www.tattooremovalofhouston.com
Fee: None, for tattoos on face and hands.
Age Restrictions: 17 years and younger for free removal of tattoos on face and hands.

Texas Youth Commission
Houston District Office
Tattoo Removal Program
10165 Harwin # 180
Houston, TX 77036
713-942-4200
Fee: Unknown
Age Restrictions: Unknown

Dr. Tattoff
5385 Westheimer Rd.
Houston, TX 77056
Contact: Carol Mendelsohn, *Dir. of Marketing*
carol.mendelsohn@drtattoff.com
832-571-2300
www.drtattoff.com
Fee: 25% off a Tattoo Removal Package–
Mention Jails to Jobs
Age Restrictions: None

Houston Laser Institute
515 N. Sam Houston Parkway East, Suite 310
Houston, TX 77060
Contact: Wayne Heintze, *Co-Founder*
kingwoodite@yahoo.com
281-789-8636
Fee: $49, plus four hours of community service for each visit.
Age Restrictions: Unknown

American Gypsy Skin Specialists
2805 N US Highway 281, #B
Marble Falls, TX 78654
Contact: David Justice, *Owner and Operator*
830-693-1025
www.hillcountrytattooremoval.com
Fee: None
Age Restrictions: Unknown

Texas (cont'd)

Permian Basin Tattoo Removal Program
U.S. Probation and Parole Office
100 East Wall St., Room P-111
Midland, TX 79701
Contact: Noelia Guevara
432-686-4060
www.txwp.uscourts.gov/USPO/Pages/
ExternalPages/TattooRemoval.aspx
Fee: $50 per session.
Age Restrictions: None

San Antonio Tattoo Removal
7127 Somerset Rd., Suite 103
San Antonio, TX 78211
210-420-8385
www.wellnessandskinclinic.com
Fee: None
Age Restrictions: Unknown

Tolbert Wilkinson, M.D.
109 Gallery Circle #127
San Antonio, TX 78258
210-495-8825
http://tattooremoval.wilkinsons.com
Fee: Unknown
Age Restrictions: Unknown

St. Dismas Tattoo Removal Ministry
St. Martin Parish
301 St. Martin Church Rd.
West, TX 76691
Contact: Jeanne Arensman
254-876-2277
http://archive.austindiocese.org/newsletter_
article_view.php?id=1431
Fee: Unknown
Age Restrictions: Unknown

Utah

Salt Lake Area Gang Project (SLAGP)
3365 South 900 West
Salt Lake City, UT 84119
801-743-5864
www.updsl.org/divisions/metro_gang_unit/
tattoo_removal
Fee: Unknown
Age Restrictions: 17 years and under

Vermont

There are no programs that we know of currently in this state, but if anyone is interested in starting one, please recommend this guide or tell them to contact us at info@jailstojobs.org.

Virginia

Make a Change Tattoo Removal Program
9540 Center St., Suite 200
Manassas, VA 20110
Contact: Rich Buchholz, *Gang Response Intervention Coordinator*
703-792-5392
www.bderm.com/about/community-work
Fee: 21 years and under, no charge, 22–29 years, $20 per session.
Age Restrictions: Unknown

East Coast Laser Tattoo Removal
2727 Enterprise Pkwy., Suite 106
Richmond, VA 23294
Contact: Chuck Powell
804-447-2300
www.rethinkingtheink.com
Fee: Documented volunteer hours for $10 credit per hour toward procedure.
Age Restrictions: 18 without consent

Virginia (cont'd)

Make a Change
Prince William County
15950 Sindlinger Way
Woodbridge, VA 22191
Contact: Rich Buchholz, *GRIT Coordinator*
703-792-7350
www.riskmanagement.departments.pwcs.edu/
modules/cms/pages.phtml?pageid=136226&SID
Fee: 21 years and under, no charge, 22–29 years,
$20 per session.
Age Restrictions: Unknown

Washington

Silver Safari Body Piercing and Tattoo Removal
Spokane Valley Mall
4750 N. Division #179 1/2
Spokane, WA 99207
Contact: Jacque Gibson Kloehn, *Owner*
509-482-3435
www.silver-safari.com
Fee: None. Free tattoo removal services to
survivors of trauma and domestic violence.
Age Restrictions: Unknown

INK-OUT Tattoo Removal Program
Walla Walla Hospital
1025 South Second Ave.
Walla Walla, WA 99262
Contact(s): Sergio Hernandez or Holly Howard
509-525-0704 or 509-525-0480
https://www.adventisthealth.org/news/get-your-
skin-back-at-wwgh
Fee: Unknown
Age Restrictions: Unknown

West Virginia

Artistic Creations Tattoos
2252 Roxalana Rd.
Dunbar, WV 25064
Contact: Adam Miller
304-744-6207
www.facebook.com/pages/Artistic-Creations-
Custom-Tattoos-and-Piercingss/187566041287099
Fee: Discounts for gang related tattoos.
Age Restrictions: None

Wisconsin

2nd Chances Tattoo Removal Program
Green Bay Laser Center
1035 Main St.
Green Bay, WI 54301
Contact: Rob Jensen, Dave Theeke, *Co-owners*
Rob@GreenBayLaserCenter.com
David@GreenBayLaserCenter.com
920-437-5277
www.greenbaylasercenter.com/about-us/2nd-
chances-tattoo-removal-program
Fee: None. Inquire for details.
Age Restrictions: Unknown

Wyoming

Re-Do-U Affordable Laser Skin Services
2909 Bent Ave., Suite 3
Cheyenne, WY 82001
Contact: Paula Ziolkowski, CLS, *Owner*
re-do-u@outlook.com
307- 632-1261
www.re-do-u-cheyenne.com
Fee: $25 per session
Age Restrictions: Unknown

Washington, D.C.

There are no programs that we know of currently
in the District, but if anyone is interested in
starting one, please recommend this guide or tell
them to contact us at info@jailstojobs.org.

Appendix – program sample forms

Once you've decided to create a tattoo removal program, one of the things you have to do is create forms to use to register clients. These forms will vary, depending on how much information you want to collect and whether your program will require participants to do community service that may require them to record their hours.

We've included some sample forms in this appendix to give you an idea of what they might look like, but you will need to create your own set, customized to your needs.

Name of Your Program
Tattoo Removal Program
Application

Name_____ Birth Date_____

School_____Grade_____

Home Address_____

City_____ Zip code_____

Home phone #_____

Cell #_____

Email_____

Parent or Guardian_____

Work phone #_____ Cell phone #_____

Email_____

- Mark pictures with location of your tattoo in a color other than black.

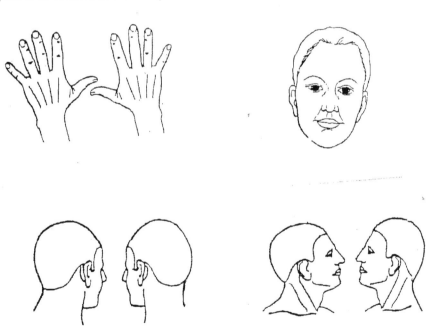

Name of Your Program
Tattoo Removal Program
Contract

Purpose:

(Name of Your Program) provides an opportunity for laser removal of homemade gang related tattoos to foster self-esteem, personal growth and disassociation from the gang lifestyle.

Qualifications:

1. Only homemade gang related tattoos located on hands, lower arms, neck or face. Tattoos must be visible when wearing short sleeve shirt.
2. **Applicants under 18 years of age must have parent or guardian permission.**
3. All forms must be signed in the presence of mentor.
4. **If under 18 years of age, parent/guardian should attend first treatment session to sign consent form.**
5. **Applicant must attend all treatment sessions and <u>complete 10 hours of community service prior to each treatment</u>. Community service can be determined by mentor.**
6. Failure to comply with community service agreement will result in applicant being dropped from program.
7. Failure to show up for scheduled appointment without canceling in advance will result in being dropped from program.

I have read and understand the guidelines. I understand it is my responsibility to comply. If I fail to comply with the guidelines, I understand I will be automatically removed from the program and placed on a waiting list.

Applicants Signature_____

Print Name _____

Applicants Sponsor/Agency/School_____

If under 18 years of age:

Parent/Guardian Signature_____

Print Name_____

**Upon completion of Program
Please send a letter to (Name of Your Program) with a success story!!**

Informed Consent for Laser Tattoo Removal

Customer's name:_____ Date:_____

I, _____ consent to and authorize _____ and members of his/her staff to perform multiple treatments, laser procedures and related services on me. The procedure planned uses laser technology for the removal of tattoos.

As a patient you have the right to be informed about your treatment so that you may make the decision whether to proceed for laser tattoo removal or decline after knowing the risks involved. This disclosure is to help to inform you prior to your consent for treatment about the risks, side effects and possible complications related to laser tattoo removal:

The following problems may occur with the tattoo removal system:

1. **The possible risks of the procedure include but are not limited to** pain, purpura, swelling, redness, bruising, blistering, crusting/scab formation, ingrown hairs, infection, and unforeseen complications which can last up to many months, years or permanently.

2. **There is a risk of scarring.**

3. **Short term effects may include reddening, mild burning, temporary bruising or blistering.** A brownish/red darkening of the skin (known as **hyperpigmention**) or lightening of the skin (known as **hypopigmentation**) may occur. This usually resolves in weeks, but it can take up to 3-6 months to heal. Permanent color change is a rare risk. Loss of freckles or pigmented lesions can occur.

4. **Textual and/or color changes in the skin can occur and can be permanent**. Many of the cosmetic tattoos and body tattoos are made with iron oxide pigments. Iron oxide can turn red-brown or black. Titanium oxide and other pigments may also turn black. This black or dark color may be un-removable. Because of the immediate whitening of the exposed treated area by the laser, there can be a temporary obscuring of ink, which can make it difficult or impossible to notice a specific color change from the tattoo removal process.

5. **Infection:** Although infection following treatment is unusual, bacterial, fungal and viral infections can occur. Herpes simplex virus infections around the mouth can occur following a treatment. This applies to both individuals with a past history of herpes simplex virus infections and individuals with no known history of herpes simplex virus infections in the mouth area. Should any type of skin infection occur, additional treatments or medical antibiotics may be necessary.

6. **Bleeding:** Pinpoint bleeding is rare but can occur following treatment procedures. Should bleeding occur, additional treatment may be necessary.

7. **Allergic Reactions:** There have been reports of hypersensitivity to the various tattoo pigments during the tattoo removal process especially if the tattoo pigment contained mercury, cobalt or chromium. Upon dissemination, the pigments can induce a severe allergic reaction that can occur with each successive treatment. Noted in some patients are superficial erosions, bruising, blistering, milia, redness and swelling which can last up to many months, years or permanently.

8. Compliance with the aftercare guidelines is crucial for healing, prevention of scarring, and hyper-pigmentation. Aftercare guidelines include avoiding the sun for 2 months after the procedure. If it is necessary to be in the sun, a sunscreen with SPF 25 or greater must be used.

9. I understand that multiple treatments will be necessary to achieve desired results. No guarantee, warranty or assurance has been made to me as to the results that may be obtained. Complete tattoo removal is not always possible as tattoos were meant to be permanent.

Occasionally, unforeseen mechanical problems may occur and your appointment will need to be rescheduled. We will make every effort to notify you prior to your arrival to the office. Please be understanding if we cause you any inconvenience.

ACKNOWLEDGMENT:

My questions regarding the procedure have been answered satisfactorily. I understand the procedure and accept the risks. I hereby release _____(individual) and_____(facility) and _____(doctor) from all liabilities associated with the above indicated procedure.

Client/Guardian Signature_____Date_____

Laser Technician Signature_____Date_____

Name of Your Program
Tattoo Removal Program

Instructions and Consent Form
For Laser Treatment for Tattoo Removal

Tattoos have been treated in the past with various methods usually causing scaring or skin changes which are unattractive.

The new laser targets the tattoo material and causes minimal damage or change in the overlying skin. 95% success that there will be no visible tattoo material neither left, nor significant texture or color change in the skin within two months of the final treatment.

Typically, two or more treatments are required; side effects are not uncommon such as:

1. Loss of normal skin color over the tattoo site, especially of the more colorful tattoos.
2. Some residual tattoo material remaining even after treatment.
3. Mild texture change or very rarely scarring in the tattoo site.
4. Darkening in the area or surrounding tissue.

For the best results in the removal of the tattoo, following these instructions prior to coming in for laser treatment are important:

1. Clean the area with soap and water and do not use creams or lotions prior to treatment of the tattoo area.
2. Use sunscreens or bandage over exposed tattoos in order to keep the skin from darkening prior to treatment. The darker color of the skin will interfere with the laser beam penetrating the tattoo pigment.
3. A topical ointment will be applied on tattooed area prior to scheduled treatment process.
4. Following the post operative instructions is very important to get the best results , please read them carefully after treatment.

If you are under 18 years of age-A Parent or Legal Guardian MUST sign this form

I have read, understand and have had time to ask questions regarding all the above material and agree to it.

_____   _____
Signature   Date

_____
Print Name

_____   _____
Witness   Date

Name of Your Program
TATTOO TREATMENT
Consent Form

The Procedure planned is treatment of a decorative tattoo, either with the use of the (Name of type of laser being used), ("Laser") or with surgical excision, using the tissue expansion or skin grafting if needed. Local, topical or no anesthesia may be used, depending on circumstances. The purpose of the procedure is to attempt removal of the tattoo or to make the decorative pattern as unrecognizable as possible by lightening the pigment pattern. There are other methods of treating tattoos, including make-up, and surgical removal may require treatment at a local hospital or health care facility.

The proposed procedure is offered through (Name of your program) with services donated by several physicians and other providers of care. The undersigned has read this entire page and agrees to the procedure.

_____

I_____, understand that the risks of the procedure include possible pain, bleeding, infection, scarring, damage to nearby structures, drug reactions and unforeseen complications. There is a risk of accidental eye injury if my eyes are exposed to a laser beam, but I understand this is highly unlikely and that complete eye protection will be provided if laser treatments are used. There is a risk of patchy residual pigment, persistence of tattoo pattern, change or permanent lightening of the skin color, change in the skin texture, hair loss, thinning or easy burning of skin and residual scar, although the intent of the surgery is to minimize such scar formation. I also understand that the risk of scarring or "keloid formation", exist in all cases, but can be minimized by proper aftercare with which I will participate. Previous treatments of my tattoos by any method may increase any or all of these risks.

I understand that this procedure fails to remove all pigment in some cases, especially with professionally applied tattoos, and the treatment may not be effective on certain pigments. Laser treatments of some white or some tattoo areas can cause black color change. Multiple treatments may be required. Total loss of skin pigment is uncommon, but may occur, although it is usually temporary. I understand and agree to my own responsibility for properly fulfilling the appropriate aftercare ("follow-up") instructions as explained by the physician or physicians who provide the service.

I understand that a picture or videotape may be taken of my tattoos and me and can be used for either teaching or publication, as the physicians consider appropriate. By my initials below I:

_____Hereby agree that such pictures or videotapes may be taken and so used
_____Hereby state that such pictures or videotapes ARE NOT to be used under such circumstances

This procedure is considered cosmetic. No representations of cure or total relief of any tattoo have been made to me, and I expect no guarantee of results. I have been asked at this time whether I have any questions about this procedure to be performed on the above named patient.

Proposed procedure: Laser Treatment of Tattoo

Physician_____   Dated____/___/___

Signature of Patient: _____   Witness_____

I have read the above as the parent or guardian of the patient, agree to the conditions and the procedure(s) planned, and hereby give my consent.

_____   ___/___/___   _____
Signature of Parent/Guardian   Date   Witness

Name of Your Program
Tattoo Removal Program

Clinic Location: _____   Date: _____

Time	Name (please print)	Removal	Orientation	Age
	1			
	2			
	3			
	4			
	5			
	6			
	7			
	8			
	9			
	10			
	11			
	12			
	13			
	14			
	15			
	16			
	17			
	18			
	19			
	20			
	21			
	22			
	23			
	24			
	25			
	26			
	27			
	28			
	29			
	30			
	31			
	32			
	33			
	34			
	35			

Volunteers: _____

_____

_____

_____

_____

Name of Your Program

Tattoo Removal Clinic History & Physical

Name: _____   Age:_____

Doctor's Name: _____   Today's Date:_____

Consenting Parent (if needed):_____

Professional Tattoo?   _____ Yes   _____No

If so, when was it applied: _____

What method of application was used?

_____

_____

_____

_____

Allergic to anesthetic?   _____Yes   _____No

Are you pregnant?   _____Yes   _____No

Doctor's Notes:

_____

_____

_____

_____

_____

_____

_____

_____   Place photo of

_____   patient's tattoo

_____   here.

_____

_____

_____

_____

_____

For office use only:

Has patient turned in consent form?   _____Yes _____No

Tattoo clinic dates: _____

Patient Name:
_____

_____

Physician: Dr. _____

Date: _____   Tattoo Site(s): 1._____

Time: _____   2. _____

                                                3. _____

Valuables Removed: [   ] Yes   [   ] No   Valuables held by patient: [   ] Yes

Consent Signed: [   ] Yes

Allergies:_____

Current Medications (OTC and prescribed):_____

_____

Are you taking any non-prescribed drugs? [   ] Yes   [   ] No

If "yes," what?_____

General Health Status:_____

Have you ever had a laser tattoo removal treatment before today? [   ] Yes   [   ] No

If no, answer the next two questions.

When was your last tattoo put on?_____

How do you think this tattoo removal will improve the quality of your life?

_____

_____

_____

MEDICATION RECORD (please check box and initial):

ElaMax5 Applied   [   ] Yes ‾‾‾‾‾‾‾‾‾   [   ] No ‾‾‾‾‾‾‾‾‾
                          Initial   Initial

Time: ‾‾‾‾‾‾‾‾‾‾‾‾‾‾‾‾‾‾‾‾‾‾‾‾‾‾‾‾‾‾‾‾‾‾‾

HOME CARE INSTRUCTIONS & SUPPLIES

Verbal: Initial   Initial

Post-op. notes: [   ] Yes   [   ] No

Notes:

_____

_____

"Post Laser Treatment" written instructions received by:
                                                    _____

Discharged by: Time: Patient Initials
_____   _____

Post Operative Instructions For Laser Treatment for Tattoo Removal

1. The skin in the laser treated area has been altered to some extent and although the chances of scarring or any other problem are very remote, rough treatment, excessive irritation or allowing to dry up would not be helpful to the post operative care. For the first few days, please use gentle cleansing of soap and water with fingers only; avoid friction or excessive scrubbing, scratching, picking, sun exposure, and limit your activities(such as contact sports). While multiple treatments will be performed, it is important for the skin to be totally healed before the next treatment. While this will often occur in one month, may take 6–8 weeks for all broken up tattoo pigment to be
removed by the body which is why the treatments are at a 2 month interval or more.

2. Leave the bandage on for 24 hours and keep dry. After that, apply antibiotic ointment daily under a non-stick dressing until healed (usually less than 10 days). If any crusting develops, cleanse with soap and water and then apply ointment like Neosporin.

3. Due to new skin sensitivity after healing, gently cleanse the treated area with soap and water and keep a light moisturizer to keep skin soft.

4. Avoid excessive sunlight to prevent discoloration on the wound during first couple of months after treatments. Bandage is better than sunscreens when outside during treatment stage.

5. Should any thickening or persistent discoloration occur after laser treatment, please contact the Program Coordinator as soon as possible, as this can be taken care of with simple measures.

WOUND AFTERCARE SHEET

In case of severe reaction in the first 48 hours from your laser treatment go to an Urgent Care or an Emergency Room.

Cleaning

- gently cleanse area with soap and water, then pat dry

- apply polysporin ointment twice daily for the first 48 hours

- keep covered for two weeks, or until healed

- apply ice packs to the treated area for 10 minutes three times daily for the first 48 hours after the treatment

- keep the treated area dry under the ice pack. Do not apply ice directly to the treated skin

- apply moisturizer when healing or dryness begins

- stay out of sun, or cover area if sun exposure should occur

- apply sun block SPF 30 or higher

- protect treated area from sun exposure for 8 weeks

- DO NOT drink alcoholic beverages until initial bleeding has stopped

- do not open or pop any blisters that might develop after the treatment

- if redness, swelling, or discharge of any color, contact your doctor

HOJA PARA CUIDADO DE LA HERIDA

En caso de una reacción severa en las primeras 48 horas después de su tratamiento de láser valla a una sala de urgencia.

Limpieza

- limpie suavemente el área con agua y jabón, y después séquelo

- aplique pomada polis porrina dos veces al día durante las primeras 48 horas

- mantener cubierto por dos semanas, o hasta que sanó

- aplicar bolsas de hielo sobre el área tratada por 10 minutos 3 veces al día por las primeras 48 horas después del tratamiento. Mantenga el área tratada seca. No aplique hielo directamente a la piel tratada.

- aplique crema hidratante cuando la curación o la sequedad comienza

- mantenerse fuera del sol, o cubrir el área si es expuesta al sol, aplique protector solar SPF 30 o mas alto

- proteja el área tratada de exposición al sol durante 8 semanas

- no tome bebidas alcohólicas hasta que la hemorragia inicial haya parado

- no abra o reviente las ampollas que podrían desarrollarse después del tratamiento

- si el enrojecimiento, inflamación o descarga de cualquier color, usted consulte con el medico

Name of Your Program
Community Service Log

Client Name_____ Phone/Cell Number_____

Date	Hours	Area/Project	Supervisor	Supervisor Phone/Cell Number

Hospital Tattoo Removal Clinic Sample Workflow

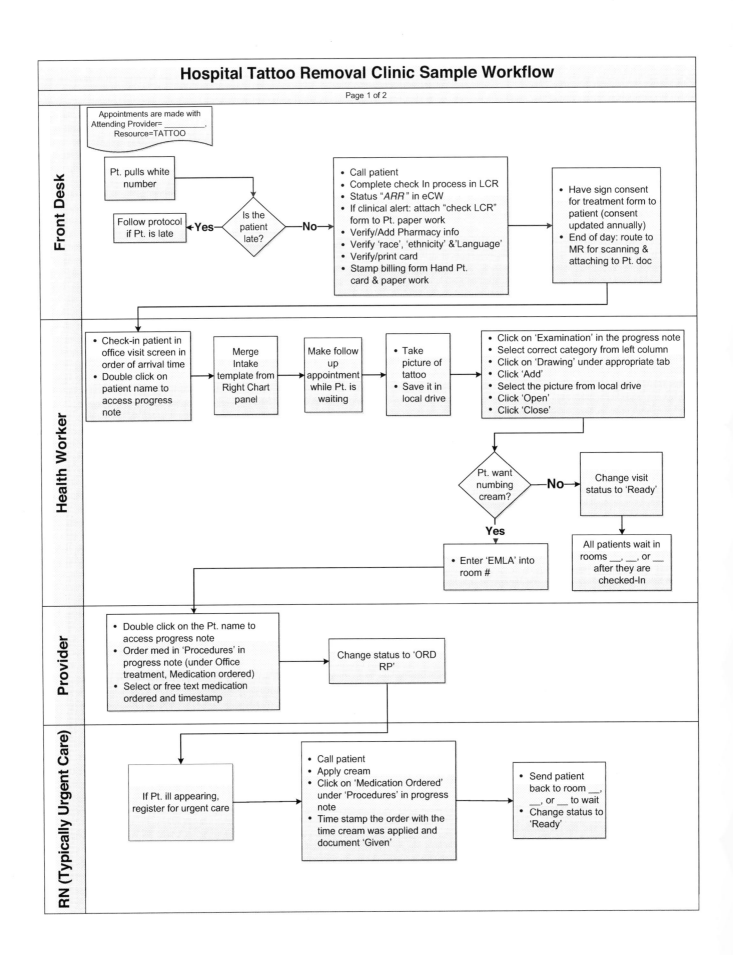

Front Desk

Appointments are made with Attending Provider= _____, Resource=TATTOO

Pt. pulls white number

Is the patient late?

— Yes → Follow protocol if Pt. is late

— No →
- Call patient
- Complete check In process in LCR
- Status "ARR" in eCW
- If clinical alert: attach "check LCR" form to Pt. paper work
- Verify/Add Pharmacy info
- Verify 'race', 'ethnicity' &'Language'
- Verify/print card
- Stamp billing form Hand Pt. card & paper work

- Have sign consent for treatment form to patient (consent updated annually)
- End of day: route to MR for scanning & attaching to Pt. doc

Health Worker

- Check-in patient in office visit screen in order of arrival time
- Double click on patient name to access progress note

Merge Intake template from Right Chart panel

Make follow up appointment while Pt. is waiting

- Take picture of tattoo
- Save it in local drive

- Click on 'Examination' in the progress note
- Select correct category from left column
- Click on 'Drawing' under appropriate tab
- Click 'Add'
- Select the picture from local drive
- Click 'Open'
- Click 'Close'

Pt. want numbing cream?

— No → Change visit status to 'Ready'

All patients wait in rooms __, __, or __ after they are checked-In

— Yes →
- Enter 'EMLA' into room #

Provider

- Double click on the Pt. name to access progress note
- Order med in 'Procedures' in progress note (under Office treatment, Medication ordered)
- Select or free text medication ordered and timestamp

Change status to 'ORD RP'

RN (Typically Urgent Care)

If Pt. ill appearing, register for urgent care

- Call patient
- Apply cream
- Click on 'Medication Ordered' under 'Procedures' in progress note
- Time stamp the order with the time cream was applied and document 'Given'

- Send patient back to room __, __, or __ to wait
- Change status to 'Ready'

108

Hospital Tattoo Removal Clinic Sample Workflow

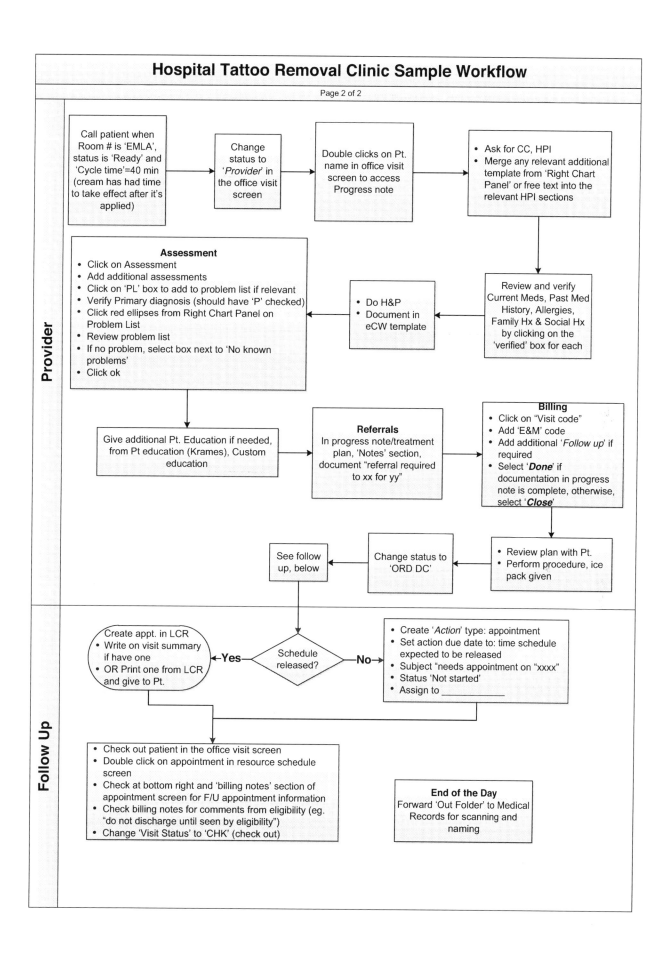

Provider

Call patient when Room # is 'EMLA', status is 'Ready' and 'Cycle time'=40 min (cream has had time to take effect after it's applied)

→ Change status to 'Provider' in the office visit screen

→ Double clicks on Pt. name in office visit screen to access Progress note

→ • Ask for CC, HPI
• Merge any relevant additional template from 'Right Chart Panel' or free text into the relevant HPI sections

Assessment
• Click on Assessment
• Add additional assessments
• Click on 'PL' box to add to problem list if relevant
• Verify Primary diagnosis (should have 'P' checked)
• Click red ellipses from Right Chart Panel on Problem List
• Review problem list
• If no problem, select box next to 'No known problems'
• Click ok

← • Do H&P
• Document in eCW template

← Review and verify Current Meds, Past Med History, Allergies, Family Hx & Social Hx by clicking on the 'verified' box for each

Give additional Pt. Education if needed, from Pt education (Krames), Custom education

→ **Referrals**
In progress note/treatment plan, 'Notes' section, document "referral required to xx for yy"

→ **Billing**
• Click on "Visit code"
• Add 'E&M' code
• Add additional 'Follow up' if required
• Select 'Done' if documentation in progress note is complete, otherwise, select 'Close'

See follow up, below

← Change status to 'ORD DC'

← • Review plan with Pt.
• Perform procedure, ice pack given

Follow Up

Create appt. in LCR
• Write on visit summary if have one
• OR Print one from LCR and give to Pt.

←Yes— Schedule released? —No→

• Create 'Action' type: appointment
• Set action due date to: time schedule expected to be released
• Subject "needs appointment on "xxxx"
• Status 'Not started'
• Assign to _____

• Check out patient in the office visit screen
• Double click on appointment in resource schedule screen
• Check at bottom right and 'billing notes' section of appointment screen for F/U appointment information
• Check billing notes for comments from eligibility (eg. "do not discharge until seen by eligibility")
• Change 'Visit Status' to 'CHK' (check out)

End of the Day
Forward 'Out Folder' to Medical Records for scanning and naming

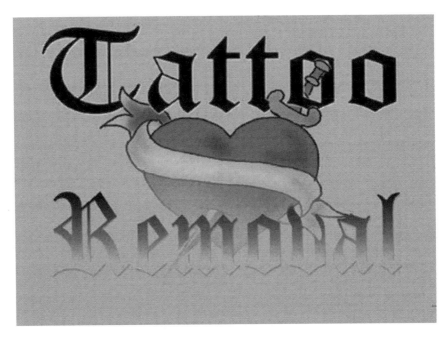

REMOVE YOUR TATTOOS
ELIMINATE BARRIERS TO:

Employment

Acceptance

Safety

We remove anti-social, gang related, and other tattoos that are stopping you from moving forward in your life.

No cost to you (community work service required).

Call (Your Program Name) Removal Program,

000-000-0000

Your Program Name (000) 000-0000

Your Program Name (000) 000-0000

Your Program Name (000) 000-0000

Your Program Name (000) 000-0000

Your Program Name (000) 000-0000

Your Program Name (000) 000-0000

Your Program Name (000) 000-0000

Your Program Name (000) 000-0000

Your Program Name (000) 000-0000

Your Program Name (000) 000-0000

Your Program Name (000) 000-0000

Your Program Name (000) 000-0000

Your Program Name (000) 000-0000

Your Program Name (000) 000-0000

Your Program Name (000) 000-0000

Your Program Name (000) 000-0000

INFORMATION ON PROCEDURE

Before the Procedure:

- Stop all skin-care products containing tretinoin (Retin-A) and AHA's (glycolic acid) seven days before your procedure.

- Do not schedule important social activities, meetings, etc., after the procedure. Most patients' skin returns to normal by the following day. However, if you have sensitive skin and/or rosacea, you can have swelling and redness for several days! Sunspots will darken and flake off in one week.

- Take 600-800mg ibuprofen (Motrin, Advil) the morning of the procedure with food. If you cannot tolerate ibuprofen, then take 650-1000mg Tylenol.

- Arrive without makeup or be prepared to remove makeup in the office.

After the Procedure:

- Do not use Retin-A, Differin, retinol, scrubs, or any exfoliatives for one week after the laser procedure.

- Take ibuprofen (Advil or Motrin) or Tylenol for pain.

- If you have swelling on your face and neck, apply cool compresses every hour.

- Apply Aquaphor ointment or aloe vera to the treated areas 3x/day until the skin becomes normal. If significant crusting or ulceration occurs, change to a topical antibiotic ointment (e.g. Bacitracin, Neomycin, etc.)

- Protecting your skin after laser treatments:

  - A sunblock containing zinc oxide is recommended, and is available through our office. This should be applied to your face every morning, even if it is cloudy outside.

  - Avoid the sun between 10am and 2pm.

  - Wear a wide brimmed hat.

Tattoo Removal

- Topical anesthetic cream (LMX 4, LMX 5)

  - Purchase LMX from the office; it is cheaper than the pharmacy.

  - Apply a thick layer of LMX4 cream to the areas that are being treated one hour before your appointment. Cover the LMX4 with saran wrap, which increases the penetration of the topical anesthetic.

- Take 600-800mg ibuprofen (Motrin, Advil) the morning of the procedure with food. If you cannot tolerate ibuprofen, then take 650-1000mg Tylenol.

- After the treatment, apply Aquaphor healing ointment 3x/day or more and cover with a Telfa non-adhesive gauze. It will take 5-7 days for the skin to completely heal.

- Anticipate 5-10 treatments every 1-2 months

Call the doctor's office for:
Infection, Ulceration, Redness, Increased pigmentation, Fevers, Pain, and Scarring

References

American Society for Dermatologic Surgery. Unwanted Tattoos. Retrieved from: https://www.asds.net/TattooRemovalInformation.aspx

Associated Press (Sept. 26, 2013). Army Tattoo Policy Tightens: No Ink Below the Elbow. Retrieved from: http://www.csmonitor.com/USA/Latest-News-Wires/2013/0926/Army-tattoo-policy-tightens-No-ink-below-the-elbow

Astanza Laser. Tattoo Removal Laser Equipment Buying Guide. Retrieved from: http://www.astanzalaser.com/buy-tattoo-removal-laser-equipment

Australian Museum. (October 2010). Tattooing–Earliest Examples. Retrieved from: http://australian museum.net.au/Tattooing-Earliest-examples

Beckman Laser Institute. U.S. District Court's Offender Tattoo Removal Program (Spring 2011) Success of Tattoo Removal Program Recognized. Retrieved from: http://www.bli.uci.edu/pubs/spring2011.pdf

Braverman, Samantha. (Feb. 23, 2012). One in Five U.S. Adults Now has a Tattoo. *PR Newswire*. Retrieved from: http://www.prnewswire.com/news-releases/one-in-five-us-adults-now-has-a-tattoo-140123523.html

Cleveland Clinic. Laser Removal of Tattoos. *Clevelandclinic.org*. Retrieved from: http://my.cleveland clinic.org/services/tattoo_removal/hic_laser_removal_of_tattoos.aspx

Cronin, Jake. (Sept. 2011). The Path to Successful Re-entry: The Relationship Between Correctional Education, Employment and Recidivism. Retrieved from: https://ipp.missouri.edu/wp-content/uploads/2014/06/the_path_to_successful_reentry.pdf

Drevno, Mark. (July 2014). Jails to Jobs: Seven Steps to Becoming Employed. CA: Lafayette, Jails to Jobs, Inc.

Grasz, Jennifer (June 11, 2011). Bad Breath, Heavy Cologne and Wrinkled Clothes Among Factors That Can Make You Less Likely to Get Promoted, CareerBuilder Study Finds. *Careerbuilder.com*. Retrieved from: http://www.careerbuilder.com/share/aboutus/pressreleasesdetail.aspx?sd=6%2F30%2F2011&id=pr642&ed=12%2F31%2F2011

Harger, Kaitlyn. (Sept. 22, 2014). Bad Ink: Visible Tattoos and Recidivism. Retrieved from: https://sites.google.com/site/kaitlynharger/research-1

Highhouse, Scott and Wharton, Ryan. (May 21, 2013). Influence that tattoos played in hiring decisions. Society for Industrial and Organizational Psychology. Retrieved from: http://www.siop.org/article_view.aspx?article=1111

Hudson, Karen L., Why Tattoo Artists Refuse to Tattoo Hands, Feet and Faces. Retrieved from: http://tattoo. about.com/cs/beginners/a/aa052903a.htm

Kelly, Annie. (Nov. 15, 2014). 'I Carried His Name on My Body for Nine Years': the Tattooed Trafficking Survivors Reclaiming their Past. *The Guardian*. Retried from: http://www.theguardian.com/global-development/2014/nov/16/sp-the-tattooed-trafficking-survivors-reclaiming-their-past

Kirby, William, Desai Alspesh, et al. (March 2009). Kirby-Desai Scale: A Proposed Scale to Assess Tattoo Removal Treatments. *The Journal of Clinical and Aesthetic Dermatology*. Retrieved from: http://www.ncbi.nlm.nih.gov/pmc/articles/PMC2923953

Legg, Dege. (July 12, 2011). The Art of the Jailhouse Tattoo. *Garmbitofneworleans.com*. Retrieved from: http://www.bestofneworleans.com/gambit/the-art-of-the-jailhouse-tattoo/Content?oid=1846463

Liberty Tattoo Removal. (Feb. 22, 2012). Inmates give back through Liberty Tattoo Removal Program. Retrieved from: http://www.capslo.org/menu-blog/51-cat-blog-articles/249-inmates-give-back-through-liberty-tattoo-removal-program

Linberry, Cate. Tattoos: The Ancient and Mysterious History. *Smithsonian.com*. Retrieved from: http://www.smithsonianmag.com/history-archaeology/tattoo.html

Martindale, Mike (Aug. 26, 2012). FBI's use of tattoos to identify gang members, *The Detroit News*. Retrieved from: http://www.oakgov.com/sheriff/Documents/TDN_082612_GANGS.pdf

Mystery of the Tattooed Mummy, National Geographic Kids. Retrieved from: http://kids.national geographic.com/kids/stories/history/tattooed-mummy

Navy.com, A Guide to Basic Grooming and Physical Regulations. Retrieved from: http://www.navy.com/inside/life-as-a-sailor/personal-care.html

Polk-Lepson Research Group (2013). Professionalism in the Workplace. Center for Professional Excellence. Retrieved from: http://www.ycp.edu/media/york-website/cpe/York-College-Professionalism-in-the-Workplace-Study-2013.pdf

Timming A. (Aug. 2, 2014). Tattoos in the Workplace, Ink Blots. Retrieved from: http://www.economist.com/news/united-states/21610334-body-art-growing-more-popular-though-few-employers-are-keen-ink-blots

United States Marine Corp. Officers Training School Website, USMC Tattoo Policy. Retried from: http://officercandidatesschool.com/blog/2013/02/11/usmc-tattoo-policy/

Vera Institute of Justice (July 20, 2012). True Cost of Prison Survey. The Price of Prisons What Incarceration Costs Taxpayers. Retrieved from: http://www.vera.org/sites/default/files/resources/downloads/price-of-prisons-updated-version-021914.pdf

Waters, Kevin. (April 8, 2012). The Tattooed Inmate and Recidivism. Retrieved from: http://diginole.lib.fsu.edu/cgi/viewcontent.cgi?article=6782&context=etd

39369216R00066

Made in the USA
Middletown, DE
16 March 2019